Talking about Spirituality
in Health Care Practice

of related interest

Making Sense of Spirituality in Nursing and Health Care Practice
An Interactive Approach
Second Edition
Wilfred McSherry
Foreword by Keith Cash
ISBN 1 84310 365 6

Spirituality in Health Care Contexts
Edited by Helen Orchard
ISBN 1 85302 969 6

Psychotherapy and Spirituality
Integrating the Spiritual Dimension into Therapeutic Practice
Agneta Schreurs
Foreword by Malcolm Pines
ISBN 1 85302 975 0

Spiritual Caregiving as Secular Sacrament
A Practical Theology for Professional Caregivers
Ray S. Anderson
Foreword by John Swinton
ISBN 1 84310 746 5

Spirituality, Healing and Medicine
Return to the Silence
David Aldridge
ISBN 1 85302 554 2

Spiritual Growth and Care in the Fourth Age of Life
Elizabeth MacKinlay
ISBN 1 84310 231 5

Working Relationships
Spirituality in Human Service and Organisational Life
Neil Pembroke
ISBN 1 84310 252 8

Talking about Spirituality in Health Care Practice

A Resource for the Multi-professional Health Care Team

Gillian White

Jessica Kingsley Publishers
London and Philadelphia

First published in 2006
by Jessica Kingsley Publishers
116 Pentonville Road
London N1 9JB, UK
and
400 Market Street, Suite 400
Philadelphia, PA 19106, USA

www.jkp.com

Library of Congress Cataloging in Publication Data
White, Gillian, 1957-
  Talking about spirituality in health care practice : a resource for the multi-professional health care team / Gillian White.
     p. cm.
  Includes bibliographical references and index.
  ISBN-13: 978-1-84310-305-9 (pbk. : alk. paper)
  ISBN-10: 1-84310-305-2 (pbk. : alk. paper) 1. Medical care--Religious aspects.
2. Holistic medicine--Religious aspects. 3. Spirituality--Health aspects. 4. Spiritual healing.
I. Title.
  R725.55.W53 2006
  615.8'52--dc22

                                                    2006001085

British Library Cataloguing in Publication Data
A CIP catalogue record for this book is available from the British Library

ISBN-13: 978 1 84310 305 9
ISBN-10: 1 84310 305 2

Printed and bound in Great Britain by
Athenaeum Press, Gateshead, Tyne and Wear

Contents

List of Boxes

List of Figures

Preface

In 1992 on a ferry bound for France, I found time to enjoy reading the news-paper and was drawn to an advert for a continuing education course that could be studied by extension. Enthused by this possibility, I managed to keep hold of the advert all through the camping holiday that followed and returned to England determined to find out more. Tentative contact with the University of Sheffield led me, with some trepidation, to start this course the following autumn. Impossible to imagine then that such a serendipitous encounter with a newspaper would be a significant step in a journey that led, eventually, to the production of this book about spirituality.

Asked to define spirituality at that time I would have talked about my faith and involvement at an Anglican church. As my study of adult learning bumped into my work in palliative care, I began to realise there was a lot more to it than that. Almost fifteen years later I remain enthused by a topic that I still cannot fully define yet continue to see influencing my work in health care all the time. I long for more people working in health care to be able to talk openly and confidently about spirituality – their own and that of their clients. As interest in spirituality grows among health care professionals, the need to articulate and examine ideas about spirituality will become more pressing, as will the need to create a safe space in which such discussions can occur. The experience of reflecting on spirituality with a small group of palliative care colleagues provided me with a unique and wonderful opportunity to think more deeply about a topic that is so often hard to put into words. Far from being something that makes people uncomfortable, talking about spirituality takes us to the very heart of what is important in health care in ways that could benefit the health and well-being of staff and clients alike.

I share these ideas tentatively, knowing that there is so much more to learn and that many other people in health care are exploring this area. I have con-sciously included examples from my experience of exploring spirituality with a number of small groups; again, I am acutely aware that many others will have had similar experiences. I hope this book will be an encouragement to others: to those for whom this subject is new, an encouragement to start talk-ing about spirituality; to those who have been thinking about spirituality for some time, an encouragement to share what they are continuing to learn. It would be wonderful to hear more about the practical experiences of other groups of health care staff; we have so much to learn from each other. Undoubtedly not all experiences of exploring spirituality will be positive but I hope many will have positive outcomes even if they are not always the ones we expect.

Acknowledgements

This book could not have been completed without considerable help and support from other people, to all of whom my thanks are due. I particularly wish to acknowledge the following: the University of Sheffield, who originally allowed me to carry out the doctoral research into learning and spirituality that lies at the heart of this book; the All Saints Fund for their financial help during that research; St Ann's Hospice and Neil Cliffe Cancer Care Centre in Manchester, who supported the original spirituality research and education groups; my doctoral supervisor, Professor William Hampton, who has continued to challenge and encourage me by acting as a critical friend throughout the development of this book; the many friends and colleagues who have shared their enthusiasm and ideas about spirituality, especially all those who contributed to the original research and education groups; most of all, my family, who remained steadfast and generous supporters even when yet another Saturday was spent writing!

A Note on the Text

Anonymous quotations included in the text are from participants in research and educational groups facilitated by the author. Quotations have been adapted from verbatim transcripts where necessary to ensure meaning is clear.

1

Introduction: Finding a Voice for the Spirit

For centuries health and health care have been understood to involve more than just technical aspects of medicine and surgery. A sense of mystery remains despite our best scientific methodology and technical advances. We no longer incorporate incantations to dead elders or spirits from the natural world, as did older civilisations, but still we are surprised by the unexpected and left with the feeling that success is dependent on more than medicine or surgery. In the seventeenth century 'the sick person was advised to cultivate a calm frame of mind and to avoid anger or sadness; he should feel confidence in the surgeon' (Tomalin 2003, p.62). More recently there has been a revival of interest in what has become known as holistic medicine, a realm of health that lies beyond measurement or technique and embraces a number of complex relationships. First, there is the relationship of the person to the self: whether, for example, a person has a sense of purpose or meaning, a code to live by and a positive or negative attitude to the world. Second, there is the relationship of the person to the natural world: a sense of wonder or oneness with the rhythms and joys of creation. Third, there are interpersonal or therapeutic relationships, including those with health care practitioners, which give the patient confidence and promote the effectiveness of treatment. Within the holistic approach, this complex web of relationships can be linked to the spiritual aspect of care. Health care professionals who endeavour to work holistically face a number of questions about this aspect of care with particular urgency. Questions about the nature of spirituality, of course, but also about the process of developing a shared understanding of this complex subject; about integrating that understanding into practice; about relating more confidently to this particular aspect of health and well-being. The multi-professional health care team is ideally situated to provide a safe but challenging context in which to explore spirituality to the benefit of clients, carers and health care professionals themselves.

I write as a dietitian who has worked in health care for over twenty years in a variety of acute and community settings. Over ten years ago, having worked for several years in a specialist oncology hospital, I started some additional work at a new palliative care centre. I began that work thinking I had a good awareness of the holistic approach and a confidence that I worked within it. My own spirituality had been influenced by my Christian faith and I knew that others would have been shaped by different experiences, but I imagined we would have much in common. Gradually those certainties were challenged by my work at the centre. Clients talked to me as a dietitian not only about their appetite but how they felt about wasting away; carers talked not only about the difficulties of feeding someone but about that person's loss of purpose and hope. These did not appear to be religious or dietetic questions, yet were clearly related to my role at the centre. My professional training gave me no answers to such questions, indeed they were never considered within a professional context, yet I was uncomfortable about failing to respond to them. While my Christian faith made me value spirituality, it provided little clarity about how to work holistically with clients and colleagues with different belief systems or even the same one! I listened hard while beginning to read and think more about holistic care and particularly about spirituality. Could these be spiritual questions? My reading suggested this was a possibility but gave few suggestions about what that meant or how to respond.

As I tentatively raised these concerns with health care colleagues, I found they too reported a new, or increased, interest in spirituality that had been stimulated by working in palliative care. Despite this interest and managerial support for the holistic approach within the centre, we were aware that our understanding and practice of spiritual care lagged behind other aspects of our work. We recognised how much we struggled when we stood alongside clients who were themselves struggling with questions about their life as a whole. Spirituality raised personal as well as professional questions, prompting us to ask about the purpose of our own lives as well as those of our clients.

In this context I began to look for an opportunity to grapple with the implications of my own uneasy sense of an inbuilt spiritual potential in every person, a potential currently often misunderstood or neglected. This began a new phase on a journey of exploration towards a clearer and more inclusive understanding of spirituality. I still do not feel an expert – far from it – but am conscious of ways in which my ideas have changed over time and how this has affected my working practice, indeed my whole life. An important part of this journey was the creation of opportunities to explore spirituality with groups of people, particularly fellow health care professionals, including the following:

- *a research group* made up of participants from the multi-professional team at a palliative care centre; the group met regularly for just over a year to 'explore spirituality with a view to how that will inform our work'
- *two educational groups* with participants from acute and primary care, who followed a course developed from the experience of the research group; each group met for four to six weeks to explore spirituality in palliative care; these courses continued after I moved out of the area and my involvement ceased
- *a Journey into Faith group* composed of participants from an Anglican church; the group met monthly for one year to explore experiences of faith and spirituality.

People in the groups began, rather diffidently, to express their ideas and concerns about this area of their life; we were mostly all too aware of our own uncertainty. As we heard others struggling in the same way we became increasingly aware how difficult it was to express our tentative ideas about spirituality in words that we all understood. We grew to trust each other and began to talk about our lives as well as our work, seeing spirituality there as well as in our work and beginning to create links between the two. Slowly we were able to develop a shared understanding of spirituality that helped overcome the barriers between us even though our ideas and experiences remained very different. These experiences influenced the way in which we worked as members of multi-professional health care teams; we had not only a greater theoretical understanding of spirituality but one that was earthed in our everyday experience. We were also developing a place where we could continue to explore the issues involved over time. As facilitator of a number of these groups it was encouraging to see the difference this process made to individuals and to teams; this book provides an opportunity to share those experiences more widely as a contribution to the debate.

Rediscovering the spirit in health care

The beginning of a new millennium was a timely moment to notice the shift of spirituality in the western world from the heart of everyday life to an ambiguous position on life's margins. Christianity, for centuries the dominant religious influence in Europe, has become simply one religion among many or none. There is an ever widening gap between interest in thriving spirituality and declining religion. Daily life continues with little reference to religion – something that would have been unthinkable even a century ago – despite surveys suggesting that many people still believe in a divine power or being – for example, the Soul of Britain Survey (Heald 2000). The fascinating Kendal Project (Heelas and Woodhead 2005), set up to test the claim that we are in the midst of a spiritual revolution, shows something of how this divergence looks on the ground. The project shows little overlap between the so-called congregational (or church) domain and the holistic milieu; the holistic approach emphasises subjective, personal development and appears to be very much in the ascendant as it resonates with the concerns and outlook of current times. Conversely, the emphasis on an external authority that seems so much a part of most religious teaching is slipping further out of favour.

Spirituality has become such a broad term that almost anything with a certain warm feeling can be absorbed within it. This encourages an open approach and broad scope but can also suggest a lack of understanding and clarity. Ideas about spirituality are left open to manipulation and self-absorption, so anything goes and who cares what other people think! In our modern pluralist society, the imposition of a specifically Christian, or even multi-faith, framework is no longer acceptable to the majority, but a clear alternative framework within which to understand spirituality has not yet emerged. The Kendal Project suggests the holistic approach is very much part of an emerging framework that includes a blurred and uncertain mix of mysticism and lifestyle, horoscopes and complementary therapies. This leaves a gap that makes it hard to talk with shared understanding about spirituality and even harder to develop a degree of discernment about this confusing mixture.

Many holistic spiritual activities emphasise the importance of health and well-being, and the changes described above have affected health care in its turn. Spirituality is isolated from other forms of knowledge and understanding that are important in health care. An increasing emphasis on the induction of factual knowledge from experience, particularly in scientific experiments, has led to a gradual separation of arts and sciences. While religion (and spirituality) is generally linked to the Arts, western health care chose to be based within the increasingly important physical sciences. Indeed, modern health care has become dominated by the scientific, medical model, itself a legacy of the Enlightenment. Vitally important for the solution of technical problems in health care, this approach is less helpful when applied to more intangible issues such as meaning or hope, or when faced with the increasingly dominant diseases of middle and older age. A growing disillusionment with the medical model of health care, explored in Chapter 2, has led to renewed interest in the idea that health care is both an art and a science. In turn there is a reawakening of interest in the holistic approach within more orthodox medicine and spirituality plays a key role in this.

Existential questions about meaning, hope and purpose are back on the health agenda as individuals look for a more holistic approach to health and well-being. Alternative therapies, eastern diets and meditation all appear to resonate with these themes to a greater degree than the concerns of conventional medicine. In fact, the root of the word for health is *whole*, recognising that it should be normal to encompass physical, spiritual, moral and mental soundness within health. Rather than being opposed to holism, orthodox health care needs to rediscover the truly holistic approach where each individual is recognised as a unique whole (body, mind and spirit), living in a particular community and able to access high-quality evidence-based medical treatment when required. Such a realignment aims for optimum health, recognising that health and well-being are affected by many things. Leisure activities, relationships and spiritual experiences, as well as physical care, all have a potential part to play. Spirituality lies at the heart of this process, reminding health care providers and recipients alike that there is more to life than the physical and material. Chapters 5 and 6 will begin to consider how spirituality can be explored in ways that affect health care practice as well as theory.

Palliative care has led the way in promoting the holistic approach within health care, considering the insights of complementary and alternative approaches alongside the very best scientific and technical advances. Yet even in palliative care, uncertainty about spirituality sometimes prevents this aspect of the holistic approach being integrated into actual practice. Attending to the human spirit, in health as well as in illness, is an essential element of the approach that is explored in Chapter 5. For example, spirituality emerges as a powerful coping force for cancer survivors; meditation and relaxation have become valued aspects of health care that affirm the spirit as well as the body; motivation, self-esteem and personality are recognised to affect health in addition to physical make-up; positive links between religious practice and health have been demonstrated in some areas. Such links between spirituality and health serve as a potent reminder that intangible aspects of life cannot be ignored by the wider multi-professional team. Ill health may lead an individual to question values and beliefs, but spirituality is relevant in good health as well as bad, an aspect of health promotion and self-care as much as an adjunct to treatment. Indeed, one American doctor compares health and well-being to a three-legged stool comprising medication, surgery/other procedures and self-care; if any leg is neglected or missing the stool cannot balance (Benson with Stark 1996, pp.22–3). The holistic approach affirms that wherever spirituality, part of self-care in Benson's image, is neglected, then health and well-being will be reduced. If health care is working towards wholeness and well-being for clients and carers, this aspect needs to be considered even though present-day confusion about spirituality leaves clients and health care staff ill equipped for that process. Our aim should be to make spirituality integral to all health care rather than an occasional extra.

Learning to speak about spirituality

Even when it is accepted that spirituality needs to be rediscovered by health care practitioners, why do we need to talk about it? Spirituality can be lost in a barrage of words that distract from what has essentially to be experienced and lived. Yet multi-professional teams wishing to include spirituality in the way they work need to be able to talk comfortably about it in terms that they, their colleagues and clients will recognise and understand. This basic shared understanding is a prerequisite for the provision of spiritual care, a necessary foundation for any assessment and action, as will be explored further in Chapter 6.

For the majority of people who do not belong to a religious or philosophical group, opportunities to speak openly about spirituality in any but the most superficial way are rare. Talk of spirituality in the past revolved around prayer or worship; now people speak rather of gardening or meditation. Perhaps all these are simply tangible ways of articulating an intangible subject. Spirituality does not fit neatly into words, while the general difficulty of expressing a non-rational concept is aggravated by the tendency to dismiss or deride spiritual concerns. Such concerns are considered highly individual and personal, and any challenge to spiritual ideas can be perceived as a personal attack by speaker or hearer, either of whom may be reluctant to start such a conversation. The continuing link with religion complicates this by creating a polarised atmosphere where it is almost impossible to explore spirituality openly with other people. One person described it in this way:

> I believe lots of people feel that it's too difficult and confusing: 'I've no idea where to start, I've read a book on Buddhism and one thing and another and that's it.' So they close the door and then they get a life-threatening illness and think 'My life's gone or threatened and I never really spent the time thinking about it or working anything out.' There's huge regrets then.

Hemmed in by such preconceptions and misunderstanding, little wonder that attempts to explore spirituality with others are few and far between. Yet clients who bravely try to articulate their ideas about facets of their lives that are more than physical or intellectual deserve better than to have their voices squashed or ignored. If, as a health care professional claiming to work holistically, I fail to recognise or respond to such voices, I am not fulfilling my mandate.

The awkwardness about spirituality is as much a legacy of western history as it is of the medical model of health care. Human rationality acquired such a high value during the Enlightenment that it became the primary way of understanding the world, with a corresponding reduction in the value of other forms of knowledge. Health care professionals are familiar with the rational language of effectiveness and evidence, but such words sit uncomfortably with ideas about spirituality that are more at home with metaphor, symbol and story. A new language needs to be learned, and the best way to do that is surely to use it ourselves as we talk about spirituality together. Health care professionals who have already talked about such issues will be more comfortable exploring them with clients. A short lecture within a programme of continuing professional development may raise awareness of spirituality but is unlikely to provide the opportunity that is required for shared reflection, where such issues can be explored naturally and constructively. Even palliative care, the strongest proponent of the holistic approach, offers few opportunities for staff to explore spirituality with others in ways that draw together personal experience and academic theory. Yet if spirituality is such an integral part of holistic care, all those working within health care need to be aware of the issues involved and sufficiently comfortable with them to recognise and respond to clients' concerns.

Initial and continuing education, as will be discussed in Chapter 3, can play an important role in helping this to happen in practice. My experience suggests that such learning requires a space to recognise and consider ideas previously taken for granted – for example, the assumption that spirituality is always connected to religion or that it becomes important only at the end of life. When these assumptions are brought into the open they can be reconsidered and challenged in the light of experience. Such reflection may lead to change (or affirmation) so that the effect on practice becomes more open and transparent. Reflecting with a group of people offers the opportunity to draw on a range of experiences and ideas from which to build a deeper and wider picture of spirituality. It also requires, to some extent at least, that ideas about spirituality are articulated. As individuals encounter other people's ideas, and attempt to explain their own, tacit beliefs and barely recognised assumptions become clearer and more overt. As a participant in one such group explained:

> Being able to reflect with people who are safe and comfortable to talk to and add bits like 'Well, I don't believe that, oh, I don't believe that.' That's something isn't it? I now know I don't believe that and that is incredibly powerful.

A forum is required where learning about spirituality can be grounded in practical experience, allowing participants to consider the implications of new ideas for their own lives and work. The use of reflection in this process ensures that theoretical concepts are related to actual practice, which in turn is challenged by theoretical concepts, thus bridging the gap between theory and practice.

What better place to practise talking about spirituality than in multi-professional teams? An individual taking part in one such exploration expressed it like this:

> I'm towards the end of my career now and I'd almost forgotten why I went into health care; this course has reminded me. So much has happened, the bureaucracy and politics over the years, and things have been changed so much. You get side-tracked and get worn down by all the rubbish that there is. This has brought it all back – that the heart of medicine is about people and the essence of medicine is spirituality.

Time spent struggling to articulate and understand these elusive ideas with colleagues has the potential to draw health care teams together in the process of developing a clear, shared understanding of spirituality. The setting of the multi-professional team is a particularly rich context in which this learning can occur. As participants reflect together, their confidence and understanding of the subject will grow and deepen. Multi-professional health care teams that develop a shared understanding of spirituality through this process will be more able to support a proactive approach to spiritual care, ensuring clients or carers are able to explore spiritual issues if they wish to do so. Greater clarity reduces the risk that offering spiritual care is viewed as proselytising and ensures there is space to talk naturally about a host of relevant issues, from complementary therapies, leisure and relationships to metaphysical questions about the meaning of life or connection with the Earth. Different practices can be brought into the open and gently challenged rather than remaining hidden. Spirituality is a sensitive issue, so this process of exploration will always require a safe space to be developed where people are able to share ideas and experiences without fear. Any group meeting to explore spirituality must provide a context that is both challenging and supportive, where individuals respect each other and are willing to listen to different views rather than simply impose their own. The practical requirements of this process will be considered in Chapter 4.

A shared understanding of spirituality

Traditionally the word 'spirit' is linked to the breath or animating principle of life, as in the word 'respiration', an innate potential within each person that can be nurtured (or perhaps ignored) throughout life. A related understanding of spirituality speaks of those elements of life that transcend the physical and intellectual, distinct yet inseparable from them. For example, Renetzky, an American social worker, describes spirituality as the 'fourth dimension' of human beings that concerns 'the power in a person's life that gives meaning, purpose and fulfilment; the will to live; the belief or faith that person has in self, in others and in a power beyond self' (1979, p.215).

Hope, love, friendship, for example, lie in this arena, contributing to a sense of meaning or purpose that inspires many individuals. Meaning may be understood as both external and abstract – for example, linked to a divine being – or internal and purposeful, related to an individual's sense of worth or self-esteem; both aspects can be important in understanding spirituality. Cecily Saunders, founder of the modern hospice movement, has closely identified spirituality with the search for meaning. She draws on the work of Victor Frankl (1964), whose experiences in Nazi concentration camps led him to suggest that not only do individuals seek meaning even in horrific circumstances, but that those who have a clear sense of meaning cope better. The search for meaning, in small things as well as large, emerges as a powerful motivating factor at all stages of life although it may become more pressing as death approaches. A sense of connection – with people, with the Earth or with a higher power – may act as an alternative practical way of understanding spirituality. When described in such terms as these, spirituality becomes an integral part of many aspects of life, perhaps not really so distant from activities such as gardening and sport.

In contrast to this broad view, spiritual care is all too often equated with religious care. Even when extended beyond Christianity to include all faith communities, this excludes significant numbers of people who have no particular religious affiliation beyond the most nominal link. It also fails to acknowledge how relationships with others, public service, experience of the natural world, art or music affect human spirituality for people with or without particular religious beliefs. A more complete understanding of spirituality encompasses spiritual well-being as well as spiritual struggle, becoming part of everyday life rather than focused only on ill health. This is relevant in every aspect of health care: in palliative care people can live lives full of meaning, even joy, recognising with a new intensity how precious life is. French psychologist Marie De Henezal describes in her book *Intimate Death* (1997) how she became more aware of this when talking to people receiving palliative care. Modern lifestyles, including those of health care professionals themselves, appear to have lost touch with this idea and rarely have space for the spiritual nurture that might help. A clearer understanding of spirituality affirms the importance of a balanced approach to life and work, and reminds people about what is important. It also suggests many ways, including non-religious ways, in which spirituality can be explored, such as contact with nature, meditation, creative activities and relationships, all activities that support spiritual care rather than encompassing the whole of it. Ways of understanding spirituality and spiritual care will be explored in Chapters 5 and 6.

Health care professionals may express their own spirituality very differently from their clients; the professional role in spiritual care is not to have answers or offer advice but rather to facilitate the client's own spiritual exploration. Although it is my basic premise that talking about spirituality is an essential part of any attempt to understand it better, it needs to be acknowledged that spirituality remains elusive. There are no clear-cut, easy answers to the questions raised, uncomfortable though that may be. Recognising and accepting shared uncertainty pushes at professional boundaries in an area where health care professionals are no longer knowledgeable experts but fellow human beings. This uncertainty reminds practitioners that who they are is as much a part of health care as what they do. The development of therapeutic relationships within health care balances technical skills and provides an ideal setting in which to explore spirituality, as will be considered in Chapter 6. Struggling with unanswerable questions about what it means to be a human being extends any encounter between health care professional and client. Being reminded of the wonder and fragility of life certainly affects our appreciation of life's value. Indeed, personal and professional learning intertwine in this area of continuing professional development with much to be gained by health care professionals as well as clients, again as expressed by one participant:

> I've thoroughly enjoyed the course, it's confirmed some of my thinking about spirituality and helped me to clarify some distinctions. But without doubt the biggest help has been to make me go and look at things on a personal level.

My own experience echoes this and supports the idea, implied in the literature, that spiritual care is rarely provided without personal exploration of spirituality.

When a particular health care team has a shared understanding of spirituality, all the members of that team are involved in spiritual care, although some may develop a greater involvement than others. Shared understanding ensures there is agreement about what spirituality is (or is not) and how spiritual care can be provided. Spirituality can then be included in routine assessment, making it clear that each person has permission to explore spiritual issues if they wish. Individuals within the team will have confidence that they are not simply promoting their own views but expressing the agreed understanding of the wider health care team. Such confidence enables health care professionals, whatever their role in the team, to listen to clients who may themselves be struggling to talk about spirituality. It also makes clearer such issues as recognising where more help is needed or who to refer on to. Providing spiritual care may be stressful, but so can not providing it where there is an obvious need; the process of exploring spirituality together helps create a supportive arena for teams to continue learning and working in this area.

Journeying together

Although it has been used as a metaphor for spiritual exploration for centuries, I have been surprised to find that the journey continues to provide a recurring theme in both religious and secular writing about spirituality. Again and again people in the groups I worked with came back to the idea of the journey: journeys of their own and of the clients they were working with. Perhaps above all, travel gives a sense of movement, ranging from dizzying speed to plodding endurance, which needs to be part of the spiritual life. Physical pilgrimage is traditionally understood to mirror and stimulate an inner journey. Writer Jennifer Lash, describing her own impulse for pilgrimage, writes:

> What an odd impulse journeying is. The external map you feel impelled to draw, with concrete, bodily movements from place to place, maybe it is an attempt to transcend a little the illusion of centrality that tends to grow about your own time and place and personality. A journey may feel as if it sweeps the skyline but the sound it makes is always within yourself. The seat of transformation is within. (1998, p.158)

Although not clearly mapped out and without a visible end, this sense of personal discovery remains an important aspect of any spiritual journey. If such a sense of exploration is part of their own life, health care professionals will have greater confidence in recognising it in others. The shared commitment to personal spirituality establishes a connection between health care professional and client such that holistic health care can never be simply a technical activity. Kearney, a palliative care consultant, describes a journey into the depths of ourselves that becomes more important as life approaches its end:

> This task requires a lifetime of commitment and effort with many false starts and disappointments along the way. What could possibly motivate us to persist with what can seem such a fruitless task? It is the sense of knowing, silent as the ground we walk on, that this is the way to the heart of life itself. Whatever our life's work may be in a material sense, this journey into depth, this relationship with soul, will be our lifetime's inner task. (1996, p.143)

Health care professionals have the enormous privilege of finding that their own journey sometimes connects with other people in a special way. This book is an opportunity to share something of what I learned in a journey of exploration about spirituality that was undertaken with my fellow health care professionals. I will draw on the experience of a number of groups, mostly based in health care, that set out to explore spirituality. I am convinced that talking about spirituality with others in this way will help equip health care teams to work holistically.

Interest in spirituality seems unlikely to lessen in the near future but I long for the time when people from all walks of life will begin to attend to spirituality not only more frequently but also more deeply and with greater discernment. This book will suggest a particular route for that journey of discovery, a journey to be made in company where fellow travellers talk as they go, sharing the lessons they have learned. It is my hope that those who take this journey will find a voice with which to speak openly and confidently of spirituality. This voice will speak a language that is shared with others, which teases out the meaning of words and silence, is comfortable with poetry, prayer and practical wisdom. This is a voice that connects with those around us, where meanings are shared, wisdom grows and the spirit is cared for as well as the body.

2

Spirituality and the Holistic Approach

Health care that is available to all, based on clinical need and not the ability to pay, was a founding principle of the NHS at its inception in 1944; it remains a central element of the vision outlined in the NHS Plan (Department of Health 2004a) and continues to act as a key driver for change in services. This is not just a question of making the best use of limited resources but of responding to the challenge of variation in disease patterns, new treatment options and changing expectations of public services. Increasing emphasis on maintaining well-being through lifestyle choices, disease prevention and the reduction of inequalities is paralleled by a debate about issues of quality and quantity of life for those who are ill. Meanwhile, health care staff are working in new ways: extended roles lead to increased responsibility for many professions and high-light the need to balance the demands of work and life. These issues are not isolated internal concerns but very much part of the wider social changes discussed in Chapter 1. Woven through these issues can be seen a renewed understanding, by health care users and providers alike, that health is more than simply care for the physical person; indeed, new health service guidance requires that people are treated as a 'whole person rather than a collection of symptoms' (Department of Health 2003b, p.6). Holism is hardly a new idea, as will be discussed later, but the arguments about understanding and using the holistic approach are particularly engaging in the current context. Although it could be seen as simply the restoration of a principle that has been somewhat neglected in recent times, experience suggests that a more radical consideration of what holistic health care involves is required. It is, of course, much easier to talk about whole-person care than to actually provide it; a better understanding of holism is only a first step and should lead to changes in actual health care practice rather than simply more words. This chapter will consider the holistic approach, why it has been so neglected within orthodox medicine and how an understanding of spirituality can be the key to its practical rediscovery.

Understanding the holistic approach

The root of the word for health (*holos* in Greek) is whole, incorporating soundness of body but also spiritual, moral or mental soundness (Little, Fowler and Coulson 1973, p.938). Similarly, the word 'therapeutic', stemming from another Greek word meaning rendering service, is taken to mean bringing to health or wholeness (Maddocks 1988, p.3). The *Shorter Oxford English Dictionary* simply defines holism, with reference to medicine, as 'the treatment of the whole person rather than the physical symptoms alone' (Little *et al.* 1973), a clear recognition that human beings have more than physical health needs, but leaving open the question as to what else is involved and how this affects treatment. Two strands, then, can be recognised within the holistic approach: first, that each individual human being comprises different elements that contribute to overall health; second, that these elements are intimately integrated rather than existing separately. The holistic approach seeks to recognise and promote a state of dynamic harmony when it treats each individual as a unique whole.

Different elements

Four key elements are generally distinguished within each individual human being. The body, or physical element, is perhaps the most easily recognised as the biological processes that occur within the human body; when bones break or cells are damaged, overall health is clearly affected. The mind, or psychological element, is also increasingly recognised, if not always understood, as the intellectual and emotional processes that form both personality and mental ability; health is clearly affected by human thoughts and feelings such as anxiety or rationality. Social elements of health can be recognised in the way a shared culture influences the health of individuals; seen, for example, in the influence of peers on smoking or drug use. Finally, the spiritual element is becoming more widely recognised as that element within each human being concerned with meaning, connection and hope. Despite this increased recognition, there is little consensus or clarity about either the nature of spirituality or its effect on health, just a vague feeling that it is important.

Any model of disease that fails to take into account all these elements cannot be said to be holistic. For example, traditionally the biomedical model of health care has emphasised physical elements, neglecting or denying other elements and, in so doing, failing to understand the total human experience of disease. While there may be questions about the exact nature of each element, it seems hard to disagree that people are more than their physical bodies and that any health provision must recognise this complexity. Think, for example, of the individual differences reflected in the varied response to something as simple as breathing. Physical disease may cause difficulty in breathing, which is exacerbated by social circumstances as well as feelings of anxiety; but the difficulty experienced will also be affected, for better or worse, by the individual's sense of hope or awareness of support. Think for a moment how much worse difficulty in breathing will feel if there is no hope of treatment, if the person blames him or herself for the problem or if no one seems to understand what is happening.

In order to provide truly holistic care, all elements of health need to be clearly understood as entities in their own right as well as in relation to each other. The physical, mental and social aspects of health seem better recognised than the spiritual element, which often remains neglected and misunderstood. Having emphasised the importance of an integrated holistic approach, it seems anomalous to distinguish spirituality from other aspects of health care; surely it should be considered more naturally within the context of holistic care. Unfortunately the environment in which we currently work seems to mitigate against such a naturally integrated approach, increasing the tendency to ignore spirituality for reasons we will consider later. By placing a spotlight on the area of spirituality, this book aims to increase understanding of spirituality not just for its own sake but in order to illuminate the whole.

Harmonious whole

The distinct elements identified in the previous paragraph are sometimes discussed or represented as if they are related but separate. Yet the very essence of the holistic approach is that each person is treated as a unique *whole* individual being. Although individual elements can, and should, be explored to gain greater understanding, it is only when they are put together that the holistic approach can be understood in its fullest sense. Imagine the same principle in terms of painting. Someone can examine individual elements, paint, canvas, brushes, marks on the canvas or paper but the picture is seen only when looking at all these together. It is this complex and integrated view of human beings, where each element is given equal value, that lies at the very heart of the holistic approach. McSherry (1983), writing about the scientific basis of the holistic approach, notes the use of the Jewish word 'shalom' to indicate wholeness and health: 'human beings are thereby recognised as a whole…where the elements of body, mind and spirit are in a state of critical interdependence which is centred on a metaphysical presence' (p.217). This connection was also made by Maurice Maddocks (1988), previously healing adviser to the Anglican Archbishops of Canterbury and York: 'Shalom, a hard word to translate into English, implies not only peace…but completeness, soundness, total well being, wholeness' (p.11). Emphasising this essential integration is vital to avoid elevating one or more element of health at the expense of the others – for example, where a biomedical approach gives primacy to the body and fails to grasp the effect of mind and spirit on total health, or the (supposedly) holistic practitioner neglects an obvious physical problem in their concern for the spiritual or psychological.

A slightly different but related danger is an overemphasis on the individual's health to the neglect of wider social issues. This may be more apparent where an affluent western society fosters the impression that individuals have complete control over their own health. Such an individualistic approach can lead to the impression that a healthy lifestyle is a guarantee of good health, and illness the direct result of individual failure, with little recognition of the limited influence individuals have on disease processes and social circumstances. Not only does this cause an unseemly victim-blaming culture, it can also lead people to an obsessive concern with lifestyle and health that seems to forget that life is for living.

Practical effect

In many ways the holistic understanding of human beings is obviously central to my own practice as a health care professional. It is very clear, for example, that I cannot consider an individual's nutritional status in isolation from their home life, family relationships, social background, education, even religious beliefs. These things affect their food choices, their motivation, their illness and response to it, and much, much more. Discussions with colleagues suggest that they too recognise the importance of working with people as whole human beings, but they also make clear that we all struggle to do so! A number of reasons can be given for this difficulty: the scientific approach that still dominates health care tends to overemphasise physical aspects of health; increasing complexity and specialisation compartmentalise knowledge; health and social care systems do not interact as they should. All these are part of the answer but I wonder whether there is also a reluctance, even a fear, of getting involved in wider issues that suggests a failure to grasp the true nature of holistic care. Perhaps this anxiety reflects our lack of confidence in this area and a very real sense of being daunted by the possibilities that can open up when spirituality is discussed.

Palliative care has pioneered attempts to recover an overtly holistic approach within western medicine. Certainly there are particular reasons why these issues are important in that area but this can suggest that the holistic approach is acceptable only as a last resort rather than an essential part of the underpinning framework for all health care practice. A better understanding of the holistic approach and its effect on practice needs to be combined with effective multi-professional or multi-agency working in all areas of health care. Personally I do not see how this will be achieved without far greater clarity about spirituality and its integrating role within the holistic approach. The process of achieving that understanding will help ensure that health care practitioners also have the confidence and comfort to include spirituality as an integral part of their work. Understanding how to recognise and work with human spirituality, previously so neglected, provides the key to holistic working. However, before looking at spirituality itself, let us consider the background to the current position.

Failure of the current approach to health care

Holistic medicine is hardly a new idea; the Hippocratic oath that remains the foundation of medicine clearly recognises that health is about the whole person and this understanding continues to underpin medical care (Cobb and Robshaw 1998, p.5). Yet, for more than a century, the empirical scientific method has so dominated western medicine that other aspects of health have been forgotten or undervalued. In particular, metaphysical ideas – for example, about meaning, purpose and hope – are often seen as beyond the scope of health care on the basis that they cannot be measured or understood. Where they are considered at all, they can be seen as the domain of religious leaders or today perhaps alternative therapists. Instead, a more accurate view would be that such ideas should not be ignored by health care teams even though we cannot fully understand them. Great emphasis has been placed on understanding and recognising diseases through their specific symptoms, which are identified by specific tests and treated in specific ways. Yet for all the scientific advances, the holistic (but admittedly highly idealistic) World Health Organization definition of health as 'a state of complete physical, social and mental well being, not merely the absence of disease or infirmity' (WHO 1948, quoted in Townsend, Davidson and Whitehead 1990, p.30) seems no nearer being achieved; perhaps it is time to recognise that something more is required.

A scientific approach

Rooted in the Cartesian philosophical view of the body as a machine, the scientific medical model views health as essentially freedom from disease. This approach has driven much of the innovation and research in medical technology that has occurred in the nineteenth and twentieth centuries. Health, it is assumed, will be restored only if the underlying causes of disease are first discovered then treated. This has led to invaluable developments in medical science: tests enabling early diagnosis, the potential to replace worn or diseased body parts and the ever increasing battery of curative medication are all derived from this approach. Less positive has been the increasing domination of the health service by acute health care where technological resources can be focused. Similarly this overemphasis on science and technology in the education and work of health care professionals means there is little room for more human aspects of health care. Such an approach requires power to stay firmly in the hands of those health care professionals who control diagnosis and treatment, offering little sense of partnership with people who are unwell or their carers. Patients are kept at a distance, becoming problems to be resolved ('the pancreas in bed 2') rather than people to be understood, while basic aspects of care or simple but effective treatments are given little value. As the management of long-term conditions and mental health exert a growing challenge to health care, the cost of medical technology is spiralling out of control. Attention to the whole person may suggest more cost-effective responses that are equally, if not more, beneficial, particularly if it ensures that we do not 'repair the body but crush the soul' (Kelly 1988).

Social and environmental aspects

A wider social perspective on health care, which recognises the importance of the environment in which people live and work, can be seen in many public health initiatives. This approach aims to treat the underlying environmental causes of disease rather than merely treat their symptoms and has helped ensure that people benefit from clean water, better working conditions and good nutrition. Again this has had a very significant effect on health, particularly in disease prevention: immunisation protects children and adults; clean water and effective sewerage systems reduce the spread of disease; and legislation protects employees from hazards at work. The shift back towards primary care, recognised by the World Health Organization as the most accessible part of the heath care system, is an important element in attempts to promote health rather than only treat disease. Widespread recognition that social and environmental factors contribute to health has led to the development of innovative health-promoting activities – for example, work in schools or with local neighbourhood groups – yet, not surprisingly, disease has not been wiped out and health inequalities remain a problem. Building on earlier work such as the Black Report (Townsend *et al.* 1990), a government-commissioned review showed that more still needs to be done to improve the health of the whole population and reduce health inequalities (Wanless 2004). Information about healthy behaviour is now much more widespread but it is clear that knowledge alone is insufficient to overcome barriers to health and promote healthy choices when people feel isolated or disempowered. This points again to the importance of those metaphysical aspects of health that can be understood as part of spirituality. Beliefs and values, a sense of belonging and hope for the future are all powerful motivating factors for healthy living.

Holism rediscovered

The social view of health outlined above certainly gives a broader view of health and health care than the purely medical model yet it still somehow misses the totality of human experience. More relevant to health promotion, there is little to meet the needs of those who are already ill or whose disease cannot be treated or prevented. Despite the increasing effectiveness of some medical treatments and public health measures, there was renewed interest in holistic approaches in the 1960s as the high cost, in both resources and side effects, of much modern medicine became clear. At the same time there was growing unease at the way in which normal events, such as birth, illness and death, were becoming medicalised so that the community's role was taken over by health care systems. Signs of this crisis in medical science were described by Illich (1976), who argued for greater involvement of ordinary people in health care, suggesting that the medical establishment itself could become a threat to health.

The limitations of the medical and social models are revealed particularly by the increasing problem of managing long-term or chronic conditions. Patterns of disease throughout the world are changing, coronary heart disease, cancer and stroke are now the major causes of death in the UK (Healthcare Commission 2004) but increasingly people are also surviving these conditions with significant long-term effects on their health. Similarly diabetes, renal disease, and even HIV and AIDS can be understood as chronic conditions; medical and social approaches have done much to treat and (sometimes) prevent them, yet they remain resistant to actual cure. These long-term multi-faceted conditions raise new questions about the nature of health and health care. People themselves are finding ways of retaining their quality of life and health, achieving a sense of well-being while living with their disease. Health care resources are limited and that is also encouraging a shift towards self-help, with new initiatives suggesting that about 80 per cent of chronic disease management can be done without significant professional help. Changes in lifestyle, joining support groups and using complementary therapies, becoming expert patients – all are part of a new, more active, patient-led approach. Not only is there a greater emphasis on self-care but this also leaves space to recognise that intangibles, such as beliefs and values, hope or a sense of belonging, have a profound effect on health and well-being. Well-publicised events such as the inquiry into children's heart surgery in Bristol or the report on retained organs at Alder Hey Children's Hospital show how health care experts can become distanced from their patients. Largely viewed as system failures, these also demonstrate the arrogance of an approach that appears blind to ordinary human concerns. New techniques or research demands appear to take precedence over human well-being and whistle-blowers are stifled or treated with derision. There seems a worrying failure to recognise that people, whether they are colleagues, patients or carers, are fellow human beings whose beliefs and values need to be heard and respected when decisions are made. Increasing emphasis on evidence-based practice, including systems that monitor clinical effectiveness, should mean that such scandals are not repeated but still does not ensure that human aspects of health care remain paramount. The holistic approach is a timely reminder of the shared and fallible human-ness of the people, clients and staff who are at the heart of any health care system.

Of course, most health care professionals are horrified at such scandals and concerned only to do what is best for their patients. This very concern can make it difficult to identify a similar presumption in more everyday situations; health care practitioners can fail to listen to the patient's perspective or impose their own views, all in the patient's best interest! From my own experience I know how difficult it is to take the beliefs of health care staff out of decisions about feeding patients, particularly if the patient's wishes are unclear. Previous experience, fears about litigation, ideas about nutrition (especially artificial nutrition) and about quality of life, all exert a subtle, or sometimes not so subtle, influence on decision making. This is complicated by the diffidence many patients have about expressing their views, something that is changing as a new, more articulate, generation demands that its voice is heard. Health care professionals too are changing and there is a move towards greater recognition of the patient's voice, directly or through an advocate. There is also an increasing emphasis on the multi-professional team approach, the view of the wider health care team contributing a broader and deeper perspective. Opportunities to discuss spirituality in understandable and relevant ways could help make the holistic approach a reality within those health care teams.

Public concerns

Public concern about health care has increased following a number of well-publicised scandals, such as those referred to earlier, and this has been linked to growing demands that the patient's voice is heard. When health care professionals' responses are somewhat grudging, people look further afield for alternative approaches that appear more in tune with their wider concerns, such as an emphasis on quality of life, links with the environment or concerns about the power of science and technology. This leads to developments that include the increasing use of alternative or complementary health care approaches, such as homeopathy, but also to the increasing use of health tests in pharmacies and other settings, the widespread availability of nutritional or other supplements and the growth in facilities such as gyms and self-help groups. This seems to fit today's highly individualistic, pick-and-mix approach to life, where people try a variety of approaches while they look for a mix that suits their own needs and situations. The growth in alternative health care appears to fill a void left by the reluctance of more orthodox medicine to respond positively or quickly enough to such public concerns.

However, this move does raise some serious issues: largely unregulated, at its most negative extreme alternative health care provides an opportunity for charlatans to profit from vulnerable ill people as well as the worried well. By the exacting standards of orthodox health care there is little evidence about much alternative health care and what evidence exists is not all positive. Desperate clients may ignore or reject effective, well-researched, orthodox treatments in favour of such unproved alternatives. With the risk of misuse and lack of adequate evidence, some orthodox health care practitioners would ban such alternatives while others point to the benefits experienced when they are used in a careful and complementary way. People coping with chronic conditions, for example, do appear to benefit from therapies such as aromatherapy massage and relaxation techniques, which contribute to overall well-being. It is also worth noting, in these days of limited resources, that alternative treatments may require less investment than medical treatments that are no more effective. This offers the potential to increase patient involvement in their own care, while at the same time reducing the demands on health care systems.

Whether as a health care professional or as a patient, I want the very best evidence-based medical care; but I also need to be respected as a human being whose beliefs and experiences will influence the choices I make about my own health and well-being. For example, an aromatherapy massage is unlikely to cure my disease but if it helps me relax I may respond better to treatment that will. Again, palliative care, where cure is not possible, has led the way in attending to the whole person and using alternative approaches where they appear of benefit, as the increasing use of complementary therapies in hospices and hospitals demonstrates. The inability to cure requires practitioners to think more deeply about health and health care, to recognise that wholeness has an importance that goes beyond physical cure and that this requires more than just a few simple additions to medical treatment. The same attitude could apply to teams working with people with long-term conditions, older people and many other areas of health care. In all these situations a more searching approach to holism is required rather than the simplistic view that science is bad and nature good. There is a deeper element to the holistic approach that should challenge stereotyped ways of thinking about all forms of health care.

My contention is that the time has come for orthodox health care practitioners to rediscover a more truly holistic approach to health care and that a greater understanding of spirituality is the key to this. Chapman restates the importance of spirituality within total health:

> Optimal spiritual health may be considered as the ability to develop our spiritual nature to its fullest potential. This would include our ability to discover and articulate our own basic purpose in life, learn how to experience love, joy, peace and fulfilment and how to help ourselves and others achieve their fullest potential. (1986, p.41)

The awareness that human beings are complex whole entities set in a complex environment is particularly important in a postmodern context, where life often seems fragmented and disconnected and a sense of anomie affects well-being. Physical wholeness is certainly not the only, or even the most important, aspect of health, as demonstrated clearly in individuals whose overall health appears excellent despite the lack of a limb or an illness such as diabetes. The holistic approach looks more widely than the body to ask what is happening, recognising the effect on health and well-being of factors such as motivation, self-esteem and personality as well as physical make-up, lifestyle and environment. Health care professionals have an ethical responsibility to recognise and respect human spirituality as a reminder that each person is a uniquely precious, imperfect human being. Understanding that people should not be defined by their disease or disability, remembering that they are human beings before they are patients, will surely open up new opportunities for partnership and self-help: 'human beings have holistic experiences, their observed disease makes the whole being feel ill and can change their personalities or their tolerance level, leading them to require a different kind of care' (Neuberger 1999, p.22). This understanding enlarges the idea of health and health care so that it becomes more profound, more whole, by transcending rather than ignoring a limited medical or social approach. Although it seems self-evident that human well-being is concerned with the whole self, and there is clearly a concern to work holistically within health care, this is not always demonstrated in actual practice. There is a genuine need to understand and overcome the barriers that prevent this approach being implemented, not at the expense of high-quality, evidence-based treatment but to its greater gain.

Challenges of the holistic approach

Integrating a holistic approach within conventional medicine is rather more radical than adding a few complementary therapies to the health care kit bag. The central tenet of holism is that people (users or providers) are recognised as fully human – a concept that can be uncomfortably challenging to ideas so embedded in orthodox health care that they are no longer apparent to those working within it. There is also a need to question wider social trends such as the isolated individualism that appears to dominate so much of life. Health care practitioners need to see themselves as enabling individuals to discover a balanced sense of wholeness and well-being within a given community and environment. The practical outcome of this approach is to encourage independence and mutual respect, ideas that resonate with many current concerns about health care, particularly linked to long-term conditions, patient choice and multi-professional team working. Orthodox health care needs to recognise its own limitations, moving away from a heroic curative model trying in vain to solve all health problems, towards new ways of providing affordable care and support that benefit patients, carers and health care staff alike. A better understanding of the much misunderstood idea of spirituality is part of this process.

Patient choice

The active involvement of patients in health care is part of a wider concern to increase the accountability of all public services, including health care.

> At the heart of the challenge for modern public services is the provision of a high quality service which meets the needs of an increasingly diverse population whilst also being underpinned by the values of fairness and equity which we all hold in common. A service which feels personal to each and every individual within a framework of equity and is good use of public money. (Department of Health 2003b, p.6)

Patient choice, based on information and accessibility of services, is seen as a key element of this equal access to high-quality health care. This principle of equity was enshrined within the National Health Service at its very inception, and choice is currently an important driver in health care provision. Increasing choice and access is inextricably linked to increasing resources and capacity, but real choice means more than simply using other providers, building more health care centres or employing extra staff. Surely real choice is only partly about capacity; it is far more about offering, always and everywhere, high-quality, accessible care that recognises and responds to the whole person in his or her local environment.

For this sort of choice to be a reality, rather than just a buzz-word, a culture change is needed to ensure that patients are viewed as whole human beings rather than just a collection of symptoms. This change shifts power from health care professionals towards the patients themselves, so that they become more involved in shaping health care. On an organisational scale this change of approach is seen in the work of the Independent Healthcare Commission, which publishes performance ratings for health care providers. New systems of clinical governance, such as the work of the National Institute for Clinical Excellence (NICE) and the development of National Service Frameworks, also aim to increase and demonstrate the effectiveness of health care and standardise practice across the UK. Choice is also about personal involvement by individuals; for example, to make effective use of the system of informed consent for treatment, people need information at the right time and in an understandable way. New technology, such as shared electronic patient records, will enable people to become more involved in decisions about their own health care. Not surprisingly, evidence suggests that people who are involved in decisions about treatments, who understand the options available to them, and take responsibility for their own health, do rather better than those who do not (Department of Health 2003b, pp.38–40).

Regular patient surveys, patient advisers and patient representation at decision-making groups all offer ways of ensuring that the patient's voice is heard more broadly than through litigation and complaints. An extensive patient consultation held in 2003 looked at all aspects of patient experience, including access, information and treatment. The result made it clear that although high-quality medical expertise is vital, it is not enough on its own, as people commented: 'I want to be treated like a person, not a number' (Department of Health 2003b, p.18). When patients and staff describe what they want it sounds remarkably like the very best holistic care:

> We want an NHS that meets not only our physical needs but our emotional ones too. This means:
>
> - getting good treatment in a comfortable, caring and safe environment; delivered in a calm and reassuring way;
> - having information to make choices to feel confident and to feel in control;
> - being talked to and listened to as an equal;
> - being treated with honesty, respect and dignity.
>
> (Department of Health 2003b, p.19)

Recognising and respecting the common humanity of staff and patients underpins such changes by increasing the sense that health care staff are in partnership with patients and carers while challenging power structures in health care. The need to support increasing numbers of people with long-term conditions requires health services to focus care at the right level and to the right people. Evidence suggests that 70–80 per cent of people with long-term conditions could manage their own conditions effectively if they had appropriate advice and support – for example, through expert patient programmes (Department of Health 2003b, p.41; Department of Health

2004a, p.36). More intensive support can be focused on the remaining 20–30 per cent whose more complex needs require proactive involvement – for example, to slow the progression of their disease or avoid complications.

A shared approach to decision making, where patients and health care staff discuss the best course of treatment together, is understood to have better outcomes as well as greater satisfaction for all involved. This is especially important in the management of long-term conditions and resonates with the holistic idea that people's own resources, including beliefs and values, are important in health care. Such a change of approach recognises the importance of building patient autonomy and requires health professionals to work differently, developing new communication and other skills such as listening and building relationships (Department of Health 2003b, p.53). Educational interventions can help health care staff to develop these different skills. For example, the NICE (2002) guidance on outcomes in breast cancer highlights the importance of psychosocial support alongside clinical care, and educational input for health care staff can help ensure such support is available. Similarly, guidance about supportive and palliative care for adults with cancer issued by NICE acknowledges the importance of spiritual care, and staff training is recognised as a major resource implication of this (School of Health and Related Research 2004, pp.38–9). Although such resource implications must be recognised, it also needs to be stated that working in this way may be ultimately more effective as well as more satisfying.

Changing technology offers new opportunities to ensure that patients' personal wishes and beliefs are known to health care staff. The electronic patient record will ensure that health care professionals and patients themselves have access to shared information and avoid patients endlessly repeating the same information. For example, a new service called 'HealthSpace' will enable patients to be involved in recording their own personal details, including their beliefs and values, faith and spirituality, alongside medical information (Department of Health 2003b, p.25). Advance directives, birth plans, wishes about organ donation and information about next of kin can all be recorded in this one central space so that it is available when needed. Such changes are made possible by new technology but reflect and support a greater sense of patient power. Just having such details on record means very little; the real challenge is how clients and health care staff alike respond to this opportunity. Clients and carers need to be able to articulate their own beliefs and values, while health care professionals need to understand the significance of such personal information if they are to use and respect it. This takes us back to spirituality and the importance of recognising the place of beliefs and values in health care. It also reminds us of the importance of listening with understanding if we are accurately to interpret what people are saying.

Multi-professional team work

In parallel with this sense of partnership with patients comes a greater emphasis on the value of multi-professional teams. Increasing specialisation has seen the development of a wider range of registered health care professionals involved in patient care. At the same time limited health care resources and changing technology encourage staff to take on extended roles and learn to work in new ways. Both these factors challenge traditional power structures within health care by recognising the contribution of many different services to total patient care. The wider multi-professional team has a shared responsibility for providing physical, mental, social and spiritual support to patients. Some tasks are specific to one particular group but others, including many of those related to spirituality, are shared. Anyone working in health care should ideally understand something of the holistic approach and, therefore, of spirituality. Anyone involved in patient care, including support staff and volunteers, needs something more, at least a basic understanding of spirituality and spiritual care that will enable them to work with people in this holistic way. Their involvement may be less formal without being less important – for example, health care assistants can lift the spirits of patients in their area, demonstrating a natural respect and acceptance as they carry out very practical tasks, an implicit spirituality that is simply part of who they are, as described in Box 2.1. Professional health care staff, with responsibilities for the assessment and planning of care, need to be equipped to recognise and respond to spirituality in their clients. Some will develop this aspect of their role to a greater extent and may become more actively involved in providing spiritual care, while others still need a more basic understanding and appropriate level of confidence. How this wide-ranging expertise can be developed will be considered in the following chapter.

The growth of the multi-professional team contributes to the breaking down of barriers between patient and practitioner as well as between individual health care professionals. Such teams need time and support to develop a clearer understanding of the holistic approach and how it will affect their work. The holistic approach will raise different challenges and ideas to a traditional medical approach, asking new questions:

In the face of death, professional masks and uniforms tend to slip and questions about the meaning of life and death steal in upon all the disciplines of caregivers. As long as this reality is denied, caregivers will never to able to listen to the full depth of each other's experiences and expectations. (Cornette 1997, p.11)

In parallel with their discussions about targets and standards, members of the multi-professional team need to discuss such wider issues as why they are there and what they are doing as a team but also as individuals. I understand these to be spiritual questions that require the team to have a shared awareness

---

Box 2.1 A patient's view of 'implicit' spirituality – the case for just 'being'

A few years ago, after a serious operation, I spent several weeks in hospital. I received excellent care from all the NHS staff but two women in particular remain in my memory. They were both middle-aged care workers. Each morning as they entered the ward they raised our spirits with a greeting and a little banter with the patients. Their work was mundane and at times included extremely intimate care as they washed and prepared us for another day on the ward. I was struck at how they switched from a teasing, at times almost flirtatious, friendliness to a professional efficiency as soon as they drew the curtains round a bed. Our dignity was protected and we were never made to feel that their tasks, although at times very unpleasant, were a burden to them, or that we were taking too much of their time. These women were not just reacting to formal training, or a protocol governing their behaviour: indeed, the consultant might have been surprised to see a care assistant sashaying down a ward to a Latin American jazz beat!

Nevertheless, they were approaching their work in a spirit that touched some of the themes raised in the concept of holistic care. We were not simply 'cases' to be treated; the common humanity of the care workers gave us a 'connection to others' that sustained both our sense of 'self-worth' and the 'hope' and 'purpose' that maintained our belief that 'life was worth living'.

Name withheld

and understanding of spirituality if they are to be considered in any depth. Again Chapman, writing about health promotion, says:

> We generally feel somewhat embarrassed to mention things like love, joy, peace, sense of purpose, connectedness, reverence for living or achieving one's full potential in the context of health promotion programs. Should we not strive to broaden our concept of health promotion to include these kinds of issues? After all what is life worth if there is no love in it? or joy? Are we only interested in prolonging life and unclogging arteries? (1986, p.38)

Such discussions are not easily started in health care practice but they play a vital part in developing both a cohesive team and an effective holistic approach. If we really believe that holistic care is important, and accept that this is what patients want, then this is not an optional extra to be fitted around more important things. If we think ourselves too busy for such philosophising, perhaps we need to question whether we are spending time doing the right things.

The place of spirituality

I believe that a better understanding of spirituality is the key to attempting to re-establish a health service that is both holistic and effective, offering true excellence in health care practice. Both patients and staff want to work in a more holistic way; discussions about the nature of spirituality and spiritual care could help make this a reality. Such discussions affect all those, patients and staff, who are working in partnership for better health care. The human spirit, by its very nature, reminds health care practitioners that people are more than just body and mind – it is also a reminder of our shared humanity, and in this area of health care no one is an expert. Health care staff, in common with much of the public, lack both clarity and confidence in their understanding of spirituality. Years of confusion and neglect about spirituality, both in health care and the wider world, have left people without the tools they need to develop this area of care in an integrated and discerning way.

My experience of working with the staff and clients at a cancer care centre suggests that considering questions about spirituality together can help develop a more holistic outlook and foster team cohesion. As a staff team aiming to work holistically, we recognised that our understanding of the spiritual lacked clarity compared with our understanding of physical, psychological or social aspects of care. Our barely formed ideas suggested that spirituality was important in our discussions about quality of life and the efficacy of treatment, yet it was hard to quantify, impossible to reduce to a double-blind research trial and potentially embarrassing to talk about. Few of us had ever had the opportunity to consider spirituality in the context of our work in this personal reflective way. Even in our well-established multi-professional team, we struggled to begin such a conversation with colleagues or clients. We could easily see how preconceptions and misunderstandings hampered our tentative attempts to explore spiritual ideas and concepts with each other but we also recognised that unless we could overcome these barriers we would not be able to provide a truly holistic service. It took time, thought and careful listening to discover an agreed core of ideas about spirituality with which we were all comfortable despite our varied beliefs and experiences. It was only at that point that we felt able to think more deeply about how that understanding could, and should, affect our working practice. Our experience suggests that the very process of exploring spirituality with other people, particularly in the context of our work in health care, was a profoundly valuable activity that affected far more than our everyday work. As we learned together, even where we disagreed, we became more confident about identifying and raising spiritual issues in our professional practice as well as in ourselves. Talking to each other about spirituality helped us talk to clients as well and therefore helped us practise in a more integrated holistic way. Two comments from participants seem to sum this up:

> I have had somewhere to bring those issues back to and to explore them within the context of the group. That increases my confidence to go out and tackle them again with clients.

> One of the big things about this group is the fact that you are always aware of how big [spirituality] is and how few answers there are … So it's supporting each other to become more confident without the answers.

It is this experience that encourages me to suggest that the rediscovery of spirituality is the key to establishing an integrated holistic approach, and multi-professional teams provide the ideal context for that process of rediscovery.

3

Learning about Spirituality in the Multi-professional Team

Religion and politics are widely considered unsuitable as topics for civilised discussion at the dinner table. Perhaps this is unfair – certainly spirituality is now more acceptable as a topic of conversation – but it does often seem difficult to get beyond starkly polarised viewpoints to begin a shared dialogue on either topic. Unspoken assumptions about spirituality make for greater misunderstanding and confusion, even hostility. Yet the groups of people that I worked with found that exploring spirituality together, in a setting where we could challenge as well as support each other, was profoundly helpful. Time spent struggling to articulate dimly understood ideas challenged our preconceptions, helping clarify what we as individuals did, and did not, mean by spirituality. As one participant says:

> My thinking has been refined by being able to talk about it academically and not just what my emotions are. The experience of hearing what other people say has formulated my own thoughts in a more structured way than I could have ever have done alone.

We came to these discussions with very varied experiences and ideas but with a willingness to listen and learn together. This, in time, enabled us to agree core ideas about spirituality and explore how that shared understanding affected our practice; later we developed a short course that could be offered to the wider team so that others could explore spirituality for themselves.

Public understanding of a private issue

As we have already discussed, although neglected in recent times spirituality is again topical as part of a more holistic approach to health care. Spirituality can be understood broadly as a concern with transcendent aspects of life, such as meaning, purpose and hope, suggesting a relevance to many issues that are pertinent to health care teams. Individual members of health care teams will be more able to recognise and respond to spiritual issues raised in their work if they have explored this area themselves, both as individuals and in teams. Hence creating and maintaining opportunities to learn about spirituality within the multi-professional health care team are essential parts of ensuring that spiritual care is integrated into practice.

Spirituality is rightly understood to be a highly personal, individual concern. Yet it undoubtedly has an impact on public life in health care, indeed spiritual beliefs could be said to affect any professional practice involving people, including education and management. Beliefs that remain tacit and unspoken wield a subtle influence on behaviour yet are inherently difficult to recognise or challenge. Isolating spirituality to a largely individual concern hinders a more public debate that could lead to greater recognition and understanding about this aspect of life. The widespread diffidence about discussing spirituality stems, in part, from this individualised approach, which is aggravated by the neglect and change referred to in earlier chapters. At one level personal spiritual exploration will always remain something for each individual but a more open and exploratory public debate would complement this personal exploration to the wider benefit. The increased awareness and confidence created by such a debate would lead to greater clarity, supporting a more robust view of spirituality. Where spirituality has a direct link to professional practice as it has in health care, this greater openness helps equip professional staff for more intense involvement where needed. Discussion with other team members has particular value for health care professionals whose work brings them into contact with people with widely differing beliefs and experiences. Again, a group member's view was that:

> For me testing out ideas with other people has been a crucial part of the process. I don't think that reading and thinking and doing on my own would

have been enough. I would only have seen it from my own perspective and that wouldn't have been challenged as it has been.

The opportunity to explore spirituality in a safe but challenging environment is relatively rare outside religious groups and these tend to have a distinctive and sometimes limited remit. Exploring with colleagues, with particular reference to a health care context, is even more unusual. Work-based explorations of holistic care often neglect spiritual aspects of the debate, while religious-based explorations rarely consider the work setting in depth. Once the barriers to discussion are overcome people may find, as we did, common threads that enable a greater understanding despite, or even because of, our differing backgrounds and beliefs:

> To me the good thing about this group is exploring spirituality in its widest sense and finding areas of meeting or questions or even differences. That means it is all right to be different yet still approach spiritual care. It's not about having one answer or one way.

Exploring spirituality in the context of a group is not a substitute for individual reflection but rather a base from which to encourage and challenge that process.

Questions or ideas raised within a group can be taken away for further reflection, perhaps when alone and quiet or in the context of work and actual experience. This cycle continues as ideas that emerge in quiet or in actual experience are brought back to the group for further discussion.

Stepping aside from spirituality for a moment to consider another area where the personal and private meet, think of the way in which health education about sexuality has changed in recent years. There are many reasons for this, not least the impact of HIV and AIDS, which has caused a radical rethink about sexual health. No longer hidden away, there is much wider acceptance that human sexuality is a continuum that may be expressed in different ways. This has an obvious effect in areas of health care such as urology and gynaecology, but is also relevant in less obvious areas such as health care of the elderly, or learning difficulties, paediatrics and oncology, where tacit beliefs about sexuality are being challenged. Like spirituality, sexuality is an area where personal beliefs and unspoken assumptions hinder discussion. In many areas of health care it is now recognised that continuing professional education about sexuality needs to help participants recognise their own misconceptions and areas of discomfort so that they can understand and support clients more effectively. A theoretical overview of sexuality cannot do this alone; time is also needed to reflect on personal beliefs and experiences.

This is not in any sense to demand inappropriate personal disclosure but rather to create opportunities where health care professionals can reflect with each other on relevant material such as their reactions to clinical incidents or case studies. As this process challenges tacit beliefs and assumptions, it makes them more open to debate and therefore leads to increased understanding.

In a similar way, spirituality should be recognised as an essential part of the health care curriculum during pre- and post-registration training because of its wide-ranging effect on health care. Simply presenting information about spirituality is unlikely to engage participants in any personal exploration; a reflective educational approach encourages participants to learn more deeply as they consider spirituality in the light of their own personal and professional experiences. Questions about who a person is and what is really important to that person balance concern with more technical aspects of health care. This link with experience soon demonstrates the relevance of this topic to many important questions about health care and human well-being, and that in turn has a positive influence on learning. For example, discussions about the inclusion of privacy and dignity in health service benchmarking can be used to illustrate the importance of respect for the human spirit in a range of decisions from hospital buildings to staff mix. Similarly, discussions about spirituality can be an important way of exploring what is important to a particular individual and therefore making decisions about treatment and care.

Basic and continuing education should really model an integrated holistic approach by building discussions about spiritual aspects of health care into the overall curriculum. Yet, as we have already discussed, such an integrated approach needs to build on a shared understanding about spirituality, something rarely available in current health care provision or more widely. Until that shared understanding is widely accepted and agreed, dedicated time to explore the nature of spirituality will also be needed if it is not to be forgotten or ignored.

Theory–practice gap

We have already noted an increasing interest in spirituality within health care, as well as in western society more generally. In 1996, the first national conference on spiritual care, called Body and Soul, attracted great interest and certainly met its aim of encouraging discussion and debate about the topic. A book, edited by the conference organisers, reflects something of the issues covered at that and subsequent conferences (Cobb and Robshaw 1998).

Interest in spirituality was booming but the organisers noted how the lack of a conceptual framework plus limited educational opportunities ensure this important area of health care remains neglected. In abstract terms the importance of spirituality is widely affirmed but in practice it seems that actual provision of spiritual care is often limited. Even in palliative care, where there has long been a greater emphasis on the holistic approach, spirituality may still be neglected or viewed narrowly as religious care.

Much published research about spirituality and health care, in both America and Europe, supports this sense of a significant gap between theory and practice among health care staff. Some key examples are given here but this is not an exhaustive list; in America, Highfield and Cason (1983) suggested that nursing staff fail to recognise spiritual needs in their clients, while a later report by Taylor, Highfield and Amenta (1994) showed that oncology nurses provide spiritual care infrequently and with some discomfort. In the United Kingdom, research by both Harrison and Burnard (1993) and Narayanasamy (1993) suggested that many nursing staff feel ill-prepared to respond to their clients' spiritual needs. Similarly McSherry (1997) demonstrated that although nursing staff can identify spiritual needs and want to be involved in spiritual care, they do not feel well prepared for this role. The majority of reported research refers to nursing staff, but Engquist et al. (1997) reported that occupational therapists also felt that their training had not equipped them to address the spiritual needs of clients. Similarly Cornette (1997) surveyed a range of palliative health care workers, including volunteers, to find that although spirituality is recognised as important in theory, this understanding is rarely integrated into daily practice.

These few examples from a growing body of evidence suggest that even where health care staff, usually nursing staff, recognise spiritual concerns, many feel unable to respond personally for a variety of reasons, ranging from practical issues to lack of confidence and understanding. My own experience, and that of the groups I worked with, supports this view. The two most significant reasons identified for this gap are the perception that spirituality is primarily the task of the hospital chaplain and the lack of education to equip health care professionals for the task of spiritual care; how well chaplains themselves feel equipped is probably also open to question! I would suggest that what is needed now is to build confidence and awareness among health care staff by exploring spirituality in ways that link theory with practical experience, opportunities like those described in this book.

I recognise this pattern of responses from my own experience in health care and from discussions with colleagues. As I wrote in Chapter 1, until I came to work in palliative care I had assumed that my work was carried out in a holistic way; it was only as clients began to disclose what I now see as spiritual concerns that I realised the inadequacy of that understanding. Talking to colleagues made it clear that, if we were honest, most of us had little idea what spirituality really meant in a postmodern multicultural society and what bearing that had on our work in health care. Those with a clear, often religious, perspective were similarly challenged when working with patients whose perspective was equally clear but very different. Where we tentatively identified the spiritual dimension at work, we lacked confidence about saying so and struggled to know the best way to respond to what we saw and felt. When we consider that clients and carers are likely to be struggling with the same lack of clarity and confidence, it is perhaps no wonder that spirituality is often pushed aside or neglected. Ross (1997a) notes that health care staff with a personal awareness of the spiritual dimension and a clear perception of spiritual care as part of their role were more likely to respond themselves when spiritual issues were raised. In the experience of the groups I worked with, the best response will rarely be to provide answers but rather to stay with clients as they explore these issues for themselves. Enabling health care staff to be comfortable listening to spiritual questions without feeling they have to have the answer was a key challenge for our groups, as it would be for most professionals exploring this area.

All this highlights the importance of appropriate education about spirituality for health care staff. There is an important place for education about spirituality in initial health care education to prepare staff for work in this area. However, I sense that a deeper and more meaningful exploration will continue to develop as an element of continuing professional education. This will build on an awareness and understanding of spirituality that can be acquired in initial education while drawing on increasing practical experience and involvement. Individuals can reflect on the understanding and experience of spirituality they have acquired during practice but are less likely to feel they know all about spirituality without ever having truly engaged with the subject. Bad practice (including ignoring spirituality) can be caught as easily as good!

Who should learn about spirituality?

If spirituality is indeed fundamental to each and every human being, then it becomes potentially the concern of each and every client; it is as relevant to well-being as to ill health, to buildings as to treatment. As such, no single group of staff working in health care could have total responsibility for spiritual care; instead it requires a shared approach involving the whole wider team as we have already discussed. By making health care staff more aware of spirituality and more comfortable with the issues it raises, they will all be more likely to recognise spiritual needs in others and respond in a way appropriate to the situation and to their ability. Their response may be to listen or support, personally or through others, but it could equally involve leaving the client in peace to explore his or her own spiritual path knowing that will be valued and accepted. As one writer puts it, 'what the patient needs from us is not psychology or theology but caring and presence while they seek answers' (Hall 1997, p.93). Ethical and professional standards, as well as human concern, make clear that the needs of the patient should be the main factor in deciding how to respond and that flexibility is needed to ensure responses are appropriate and timely. Time to explore our own spirituality and its effect on our work will surely help ensure that our response is less cluttered by personal issues.

Every member of a health care team requires the basic understanding of what spirituality is, and how that might be recognised and responded to within health care settings. A smaller number of staff, perhaps only one or two, may develop a specific role as co-ordinator or adviser for spiritual care for a team or area – for example, taking a lead on documentation and assessment, ensuring that new staff receive training and more established ones remain up to date. In between these two positions, a number of staff may elect to explore this area in greater depth, becoming more aware of their own spirituality and that of their clients. In some areas of health care, such as oncology, palliative care or chronic disease management, the motivation to understand spirituality more deeply may be greater but there should perhaps be individuals in every area of health care who elect to explore this area of care more fully. Any member of staff could choose to become more active in this way but there are particular reasons why professional health care staff should understand spirituality better. Spirituality can be seen to be more formally linked to their role, particularly in assessment and care planning. Again, nursing staff are often assumed to have a particular duty to be involved in spiritual care but there appears no reason to suppose that other health care professions could not be involved in a similar way, especially in areas where there is a strongly multi-professional approach. This approach increases the resources available, in terms of understanding and experience, and ensures spirituality is integrated into the total package of health care. It also offers mutual support in an area that can be emotionally demanding and where support may be lacking. The research that supports NICE guidelines on supportive and palliative care for adults with cancer includes no studies that discuss spiritual support for staff (King's College London 2004, p.175).

Without wider active involvement there remains the risk that something as complex and difficult to articulate as spirituality will be missed, perpetually viewed as someone else's role with no one feeling any real sense of ownership or expertise in this area and the potential to cause harm to vulnerable clients. Developing a shared understanding of spirituality and spiritual care offers an opportunity to help the multi-professional team recognise its shared responsibility in this area and creates a sense of ownership about spirituality across the team. Shared understanding enables effective communication and supports consistent working practices that help ensure spiritual care is timely and appropriate. Although relevant to all health care teams, those involved in the management of long-term conditions or palliative care may be more ready to consider spirituality in depth and recognise their own involvement in this area. Long-standing involvement with a single patient group tends to offer greater opportunities to build relationships that provide an appropriate context to discuss issues such as hope or meaning and purpose. Again, although involvement in this process is relevant to all team members, individuals will be involved in differing ways and to differing degrees.

Nursing and other health care professionals

Within the multi-professional health care team, as already discussed, nursing has traditionally emphasised the holistic approach, including the importance of spirituality. The sustained contact many nurses have with patients ensures they are particularly well placed to recognise spiritual needs and develop relationships within which spiritual care can be provided. Spirituality and the provision of spiritual care is written into the nursing code of conduct, yet as in the rest of health care, actual practice does not always reflect this ideal, as discussed earlier. Nurses have, nevertheless, played a key role in the renewed interest in spirituality, as can be seen in the growing number of books, conferences and research articles on this subject in the nursing press as well as the growing body of nurse-led research on this topic. Even the recognition that spirituality is not actually well integrated into practice can be seen as an important step forward, a place from which to build a more integrated approach. On the opposite side of this debate is the concern that the wider involvement of nursing and other health care staff in providing spiritual care without proper understanding of all that involves, will be harmful. The response to such concerns is surely to improve understanding rather than to exclude an invaluable resource.

If spirituality needs a team approach, then other health care professionals besides nurses need to become actively involved in considering this subject. Twycross and Lack (1990, pp.2008–9) provide a framework to help medical staff recognise spiritual concerns but suggest that people are more likely to discuss such issues with other members of the team or with friends and relatives. The increasing involvement of a range of allied health professionals in patient care suggests other key groups to involve in the debate about spirituality and this certainly reflects my experience as a dietitian working in palliative care. The groups that I worked with involved occupational therapists and dietitians as well as medical and support staff, including volunteers. Despite a mischievous suggestion that physicians should be prescribing religious activities (Sloan *et al.* 2000) and discussion by occupational therapists about the place of spirituality in rehabilitation (for example, in the research by Engquist *et al.* 1997 referred to earlier), little seems to have been written on this subject from the perspective of other professions. This may change as interest in spirituality increases and it becomes more widely recognised as an integral part of health care for professional groups across the whole spectrum. There are particular incentives to explore spirituality in the care of people with long-term conditions, including elderly care, mental health care and palliative care, where contact is likely to be prolonged as well as raising pertinent concerns. Research by the Methodist Housing Association (MHA) Care Group is looking at two neglected areas of spirituality – those of older men and of people with dementia (MHA Care Group 2005). Birth is another time when questions about spirituality may be raised, either in wonder at new life or pain at loss of hope or life, and there is growing interest in spirituality within midwifery (Hall 2000).

Involving chaplaincy services

The role of the chaplain as part of the health care team also needs to be considered carefully. In 1991, the Patients' Charter (Department of Health 1991) stipulated that respect for multi-faith religious belief was a fundamental right, to be considered alongside the right to privacy and dignity. This need for respect, plus revised guidelines on spirituality and spiritual care (Department of Health 2003a), has stimulated a review of the nature and delivery of expanding chaplaincy services. There is an important role for chaplains in ministry to those with specific religious needs from different faith communities, particularly as these needs may become more pressing during periods of illness. Such specific beliefs and practices remain important to many individuals even where their connection to a particular religious group appears superficially quite nominal. Some of this support will be provided directly by chaplains or chaplaincy volunteers, but greater awareness will help the wider health care team to recognise the scope and variety of religious needs. Many chaplains also recognise staff support as a key element of their role, and the provision of staff counselling and pastoral care from someone slightly outside the hospital structure can be a very valuable resource. Health care chaplains, then, tend to be well regarded as a valuable asset without there necessarily being a real understanding of their role or integration at an organisational level. For example, chaplaincy services may be marginalised within health care trusts and are rarely involved in business planning or normal service monitoring (Orchard 2000).

The tension between a central and marginal role will not be unfamiliar to clergy in parish and other settings (Redfern 1999, pp.38–9). Being on the edge of the organisation can be helpful for clergy working in health care – for example, when supporting staff or clients – but should not exclude them from decision-making processes or organisational systems. While a degree of neutrality can be a positive aspect of chaplaincy services, it should not lead to their isolation from everyday activity within health care organisations. It is clear that if spirituality becomes more integrated into holistic care for all clients and carers then it also becomes more visibly the task of the whole health care team as we have discussed. Rather than being viewed as exclusive providers of spiritual care, chaplaincy staff of all denominations and faiths have much to offer the multi-professional team that chooses to reflect on spirituality and spiritual care. Chaplains themselves will also have much to gain as they explore these issues with other members of the health care team.

A chaplain might appear the obvious choice to co-ordinate spiritual care, including promoting the inclusion of spirituality at a strategic level and taking a lead on staff training about spirituality. Indeed this role may usefully be linked to chaplaincy services at an organisational level, although there are unlikely to be enough chaplains to enable every health care team to use a chaplain in this way. Most chaplains are very familiar with the debates about spirituality and religion and are actively involved in staff training – for example, about the needs of different faith communities – as well as working to increase awareness of personal spirituality among staff. In many areas, the spiritual care of staff is also traditionally viewed as the chaplain's role and provides an invaluable service that includes counselling and bereavement support. Pattison (2001, p.39) suggests that the contribution of chaplains to spiritual care may be more helpful if they remain clear about the distinctiveness of their religious identity and discipline while being open to discussing other ideas and traditions. Chaplaincy services may be seen as too religiously partisan by both staff and patients for the role of co-ordinator. There also remains a risk that chaplains will continue to be viewed as spiritual experts in a way that reinforces the tendency to hand over spiritual issues to the chaplain rather than encouraging wider team involvement. Perhaps a better approach is to ensure that chaplaincy services are involved with other members of the health care team in exploring spirituality and spiritual care, while different members of the health care team adopt the co-ordinating role for the team.

Involving the wider team

Involving clinical and other staff, such as chaplains, in debates and training about spirituality mirrors the good practice of involving the whole team in the actual provision of spiritual care. However, this leaves open the question of how widely each team extends and there may be practical difficulties about involving team members who work across several teams. As a dietitian working in several areas I was glad to be involved in discussions about spirituality in one specific team but I would never have been able to become involved in such discussions if they were occurring in all the areas where I worked. Perhaps some training and awareness-raising needs to occur at the level of the wider organisation to enable the extended team to be realistically involved in spiritual care.

Again within the wider team support staff, such as catering and cleaning staff who provide basic care, are often neglected when thinking about spirituality. This is to forget that the health care assistant who listens while washing a patient may understand more of what makes that person tick than the doctor who sees the patient briefly at a formal ward round. Carrying out the most prosaic activities in a manner that demonstrates respect and humanity surely implies a great deal about practical spirituality even where those involved cannot easily explain that connection. Although they may not articulate their understanding of spirituality, health care staff who provide the most basic care still play a significant role in spiritual care, as the reflection in Box 2.1 (p.39) suggests. Here an unspoken spirituality was implicit in the way that everyday tasks such as washing, feeding and dressing were carried out, and helped to create an environment where the human spirit could flourish. Such influences need to be recognised and included in the overall understanding of spiritual care. The involvement of volunteers could also be included here; again they are generally active on the margins of health care teams but may still play a significant part in patient support, sometimes more available to listen or be with people than busy professional staff. Such members of the wider health care team make a vital contribution to the atmosphere of any health care environment and therefore to client well-being. By simply giving someone positive attention throughout the most mundane activity, they demonstrate respect and practical care that can help raise the spirits and restore a sense of worth; a little fun and laughter help too. These contributions to spiritual or holistic care often receive little recognition, so that the team as a whole misses this perspective while the individuals involved miss the support of other team members. They need to operate within the same spiritual framework as the rest of the team and will have their own needs for support and training. Indeed their needs may be even greater than those of health care professionals, whose previous training should have equipped them with basic coping mechanisms for dealing with difficult questions and who may well have other systems of professional support and supervision. The empirical study in Belgium referred to earlier reported that volunteers experienced significant spiritual distress in their work yet did not see the multi-professional team as an appropriate forum for discussing their personal or spiritual needs (Cornette 1997, p.10).

The difficulty of articulating spirituality

Exploring spirituality in the context of a group demands, to a significant degree, that ideas and experiences about spirituality are articulated, something that is often unfamiliar, difficult and uncomfortable. An early inquiry into whole-person medicine described it in this way:

> How can one person know what another person means by the word [spirit]? With people with different cultures, classes and religious affiliations there are bound to be markedly different interpretations attached to the word, leading to misunderstanding and confusion. The Tower of Babel. Many people have thought so little about the subject and only have a rather diffuse idea as to what they mean themselves when they use the word, let alone what you mean when they hear you use the word. (Reason and Heron 1985, p.52)

There are a number of reasons why spirituality can be so difficult to talk to other people about. Superficially, as we have already discussed, the common view of spirituality as highly personal means that people are reluctant to discuss it in public, fearing either to intrude or be ridiculed. While older patients may retain some religious language and understanding, younger people particularly often have little shared vocabulary with which to discuss religion or spirituality (Davie and Cobb 1998, p.97). Furthermore, in a context where a scientific view of health care is dominant, metaphysical ideas may be marginalised or devalued, and staff or patients may be cautious about voicing ideas about spirituality in case these are not taken seriously or are dismissed as irrelevant. For health care professionals there may be the added concern about opening a proverbial can of worms by raising questions to which we do not know the answers. As time goes on a simple lack of practice perpetuates this difficulty of not knowing quite what to say about spirituality or how to say it. The historical link between spirituality and religion aggravates this confusion with both a struggle to understand a spirituality that is not necessarily religious and a fear of being suspected of proselytising. Conversely the polarisation of views around religion rubs off on spirituality to create an atmosphere that encourages people to argue and take sides, something that rarely helps people to listen to each other. In an atmosphere of busyness, where words are so difficult to find and the consequences of getting it wrong potentially so uncomfortable, it is easier to say nothing.

I suspect that underlying all these factors is an inherent sense, perhaps an accurate one, that spirituality is in some sense beyond words. David Jenkins, a former Bishop of Durham, referred to spirituality at a conference I attended as a 'slippery word' implying that it is difficult to fully grasp a meaning that seems to shift and change (1997). For me, this echoes the description of spirituality, used in Cornette's (1997) study, as a 'horizon which is always moving on' (p.7). To recognise the difficulties inherent in talking about spirituality is one thing, a useful reminder that this is a complex and many-layered subject; to blithely and continually extend our understanding of what spirituality is all about heads dangerously towards ever greater muddle and confusion. Pattison points out that spirituality is beginning to 'function like intellectual polyfilla, changing shape and content conveniently to fill the space its users devise for it' (2001, p.37). In this situation, educational groups can bring a helpful challenge, encouraging discernment and providing a wider resource within which to explore ideas about spirituality. Apart from the real danger of spirituality simply becoming a bland generalisation that suits no one, it is not impossible that a spiritual feeling or experience profoundly helpful to one individual may be equally unhelpful to another or to the wider community. Wakefield quotes the example, perhaps rather extreme, that Hitler was understood to have a powerful spirituality yet one that is clearly recognised to have been harmful in the wider world (1983, p.362). In our own group discussions there were, at times, obvious tensions between individuals with very different views about personal spirituality. These differences were obvious from the beginning but it was only as the group became accepted as a safe space that people were able to talk openly about their differences and consider how to cope with them in the shared health care team. Greater clarity about the nature of spirituality, including the understanding that there are boundaries to what it is and is not, was a helpful element of these discussions.

I would be very reluctant to suggest that spirituality can ever be neatly pinned down into an adequate form of words, nor indeed can it ever be fully known. However, words are one of our main tools of communication; talking about spirituality requires us to learn a new and different language, using metaphors and stories rather than measurements and symptoms. It also encourages a helpful focusing as we struggle to articulate unfamiliar ideas and barely recognised insights. Of course, this is a salutary reminder of how patients and carers can feel as they get caught up in the health care systems with which we are so familiar. Health care professionals become vulnerable as they struggle with this new language and the essential human questions being raised. This can be a very challenging, even painful, process and certainly reminds us of our humanity. Exploring spirituality with others requires careful attention to what people are saying, struggling to understand what they mean rather than just hearing the words they are using. Such meaning is often complex and many layered, even contradictory (Usher 1993, p.172), particularly as people's own ideas are evolving. Health care professionals need to be aware that clients may refer to spirituality through metaphors, pictures or symbols; even jokes and throwaway lines can be used to raise a topic that is hard to talk about. If we are not aware of this, such references will be lost and may not occur again.

Many of the people involved in the groups I organised expressed a feeling that they were somehow not the right sort of person to be involved in a discussion about spirituality. Further inquiry suggested that this feeling stemmed from their perception that they did not understand spirituality clearly enough or that they were not religious enough. However, these causes were compounded by the difficulty of having to articulate their ideas about spirituality in words. As the groups I worked with continued and these feelings about spirituality were shared, we became more comfortable with our own incomplete understanding and inarticulateness. Individuals described how difficult this issue could be in encounters with clients, recognising how both they and their clients struggled to find the words to talk about spirituality accurately and with common understanding. At first, groups needed time to overcome these feelings but as we learnt to trust each other we were more able to express and tease out our ideas about spirituality. This process helped us understand our own ideas better, as well as those of other group members, as these two quotes suggest:

> For me, testing and feeling out ideas with other people has been a crucial part of the process.

> It's been good to have such a mix of people because often one tends to talk to like-minded people about your views in this area which doesn't give you the same challenge.

What we held in common, despite our very different faith and world-views, became clearer as the groups continued. We found that exploring together in a safe setting on a regular basis helped overcome our anxieties about this topic; we became more comfortable about exploring with each other. In fact, we began to find the process of talking about spirituality both liberating and absorbing, certainly worth the effort involved. Although it seems contrary to the idea that spirituality is integral to all of health care to focus on it in this way, our experience suggested it was helpful to explore spirituality specifically. We turned the spotlight on spirituality, in a sense, in order to reintegrate it into our health care practice with greater understanding. Having done that, we recognised deep within ourselves that spirituality is not an outdated eccentricity or an unnecessary luxury; it is an integral part of all health care practice, more about who we are than what what we do. Exploring spirituality in the context of health care practice promises benefits for health care professionals and their clients, something that will be explored in later chapters.

The whole-team approach

A multi-professional, whole-team approach is central to the integration of spirituality within holistic health care including the provision of effective spiritual care. Hence the importance of creating opportunities for members of the health care team to reflect together on the nature of spirituality and spiritual care. Rather than educating only a small number of spiritual specialists, this approach ensures that spirituality is considered in a more consistent and integrated way by the whole team. By reflecting on a range of practice-based experiences and ideas, the team is able to create and own a wider and deeper picture of spirituality that is embedded in its members' own experience. This approach both reinforces and requires a sense of shared responsibility for spirituality where the contribution of each team member is valued and respected.

Indeed spirituality may help with this as it cuts across increasing specialisation and separation of tasks.

Rather than spirituality becoming an additional task, this exploration should help team members recognise it as a profound influence on many of the basic activities that make up their daily work. Our understanding of what it is to be human affects the way we treat our clients in the most mundane and intimate of tasks. A shared understanding of spirituality adds depth to discussions – for example, about one of the team's clients who is struggling with treatment or diagnosis or in the wake of a particularly difficult death, events that happen all the time in both primary and secondary care. The recognition that spirituality is part of our shared humanity raises new questions when team members talk about coping with the stress of working with people who are seriously ill; questions that touch on our own sense of meaning or hope as well as that of our clients. Public acknowledgement that it is just not possible to sort out all the problems of human health, body, mind or spirit, helps new staff as they learn to cope with their own feelings about failure and loss. An understanding of spirituality and spiritual care, and the process leading to that understanding, adds something to these team processes, places them in a wider context or perhaps helps them occur at a greater depth.

Although a whole-team exploration of spirituality can help build team cohesion and support, it does require an effective working team. An exploration of spirituality should not be seen as the way to resolve difficulties within the team. Malfunctioning teams, already affected by friction or in-fighting, will not be ready to start a discussion that requires people to be open about their personal beliefs and values. Such a setting would be wholly inappropriate for so personal a process and would risk causing damage to individuals and the team.

Personal and professional

We have already discussed how spirituality can be understood as both a personal and a public concern in health care, and recognised that a shared understanding of spirituality is essential for all members of health care teams that purport to offer holistic care. While any discussion of spirituality touches on issues that are undoubtedly personal, this is essentially an exploration that aims to affect working practice to the benefit of patients as well as individual members of staff and their employers. It is one thing to discuss spirituality in theoretical terms, quite another to explore in a more professionally demanding way, especially when that may also have personal implications. Individuals with a clear grasp of their own spirituality (however they understand that spirituality) may find this as difficult as those with a less clearly committed viewpoint, while other staff may simply not see the relevance of this area of learning for their work at all. For these reasons, opportunities to learn about spirituality should be available to all those involved in the wider multi-professional team, although full participation in such personal educational opportunities must remain voluntary. Some will want to learn about this topic for its own sake, perhaps because of a previous experience or particular interest; others may be more motivated to learn as they recognise its relevance to their working practice or personal experience; yet others will remain resistant to learning anything more than a basic understanding of the topic. Actively supporting the involvement of the wider team is complex, especially with the need to build a shared understanding between staff with very different experiences and backgrounds. Spirituality is certainly not only the province of senior or professional team members; the whole team is involved in this area of care, including ancillary staff and volunteers, yet their roles will be different. While some basic awareness of spirituality is surely appropriate for all health care staff, individual team members should be able to learn in different ways and to differing degrees depending on their actual involvement and role.

Reiterated in much of the writing about spiritual care is the impression that providing spiritual care is enhanced by personal understanding and experience of spirituality. We have already seen how health care raises many questions about life yet provides few settings in which to reflect openly on these questions. The personal beliefs and values of a health care worker may be challenged by encounters with suffering and joy – for example, by the unexpected death of a patient or, equally, by a patient who transcends the difficulties of his or her condition. Such occurrences may create moments when individual health care professionals are particularly open to learning about this complex and personal issue. Of course, health care staff may still choose to ignore such thoughts and questions when they are raised by encounters with patients. Sometimes this is a necessary protection but at other times individuals and teams may find it helpful, with appropriate support, to consider them within discussions about spirituality. The process of exploring spirituality offers potential benefits for any health care professional's own personal and professional development. The increased confidence and understanding about spirituality that this brings means that patients' spiritual concerns can also be responded to appropriately and that too brings health care benefits. Clinical supervision offers one helpful opportunity for an individual health care professional to reflect about these issues with another individual. Reflecting with a group of colleagues has the added advantage of a wider range of ideas and experiences as well as more support; varied ideas may create some tension but do lead to a more robust and rounded understanding. When that group is an established team and this process leads to a shared understanding of spirituality, this will affect the activity of the team as well as creating a more cohesive team in the way this group member describes:

> I now understand a bit more about how other people in the team tick and that puts a different dimension on the working relationship. It's obviously a big part of people's belief and value system but you don't always talk about it. It is quite useful to have that connection.

Boundaries

Health care professionals operate within boundaries that are intended to protect both themselves and their clients. Vulnerable clients must be protected from mental, emotional or physical abuse; vulnerable health care professionals must be protected from burning out when the emotional and physical demands upon them become too great. Increased understanding of spirituality and spiritual care ensures that clients and health care professionals alike are recognised as unique, whole human beings, an enriching process for both. The concerns about meaning and values that lie at the heart of spirituality and spiritual care cannot easily be understood without recognising that health care professionals and their clients share a common humanity. Yet that understanding needs to remain within professional boundaries, despite the tensions this might cause, in order to avoid harm to either side. Spiritual care, particularly at the end of life, appears to require that professional boundaries are sometimes transcended, yet this will have a cost that must also be taken into account. The provision of spiritual care will have physical costs, such as staff time and energy, but perhaps more important are the emotional and spiritual costs of engaging with people in this way. Individuals may find their own values or beliefs challenged, perhaps in a way that is ultimately enriching but also disturbing. Understanding spirituality in health care better is intended to be a practical response to such tensions rather than adding to them, a positive contribution to set against the costs involved. Exploring spirituality in the ways outlined in this book will give those who take part greater confidence about the provision of spiritual care. It will also make people more aware of the need for self-care in terms of spirituality, encouraging opportunities to nurture their own spirituality and thus reduce stress. Greater personal awareness of spirituality may help health care professionals recognise, and limit, some of the costs outlined above.

Risk and reward

Exploring spirituality with groups of health care staff demonstrated the inevitability of linking personal and professional in this area more clearly than I expected. Rather than simply giving new information, these were specific opportunities to consider theoretical ideas, old and new, in the light of personal experience. The safe space we were able to create became a place where we could tentatively explore our own questions as well as those of our patients. The aim of the groups I worked with, agreed with the participants, was 'to explore our own spirituality with a view to how that informs our work'. As we explored together, ideas that had been quietly taken for granted were recognised and reconsidered while new ideas about spirituality were challenged by our varied personal experiences. It was only as we worked towards a shared understanding of spirituality that we were able to discuss more constructively the practical provision of spiritual care in our places of work. We increasingly saw how being more comfortable with our own spirituality, whatever form that took, was helpful in our work; greater clarity enabled us to recognise when patients were expressing spiritual concerns; greater comfort and confidence helped us respond appropriately. We then found it easier not to shy away from such issues but began to see them as simply another element of our work, something to listen to and consider. We recognised our role in this process as companion rather than expert and began to see how being unaware of our own spirituality could be a hindrance to that role. Knowing that we could go back and explore our own thoughts and feelings about spirituality in the group helped us cope when our contact with clients raised difficult or painful feelings.

Exploring spirituality with other people carries an in-built risk just because this area is so central to one's personality. My personal belief system may be somewhat submerged but it is a core part of who I am and how I view myself: when I focus attention on spirituality I look deep within myself and doing this with others poses a significant risk to my self-image. Talking about spirituality, then, particularly where ideas are being formed or revised, occurs best in an atmosphere of mutual trust and respect. Being open to learn from others, to be challenged by what others are saying or by their experiences, is a prerequisite for an exploration that may lead to a greater understanding of myself as well as other people and the issues involved. If the group goes well, my spirituality will grow and develop as I become more confident about this area of life but if such a central element of who I am is treated harshly then it is potentially damaging, even destructive. For these reasons the context and educational approach of such groups is very important and will be explored in detail in the next chapter.

There is yet another risk associated with spirituality in a health care setting that I now want to explore further. If spirituality is essentially about what it is to be human, then health care professionals and patients alike struggle with the issues and questions that it raises. There is a sense of equity about any discussion of spirituality; no one has all the answers; most people recognise that they are out of their depth in this area. Michael Kearney, in his book *Mortally Wounded* (1996), talks about the need for health care to recognise that it cannot always be victorious in the battle with suffering and death. Palliative care provides a poignant reminder that this is true in any aspect of health care but spirituality provides a slightly different challenge to our professional pride. We simply do not have the right or ability to sort out anyone's life in this way, particularly when we can hardly resolve our own spiritual concerns. This is not to discount the professional expertise of any member of the health care team but simply to recognise its limitations; spirituality highlights the fact that within our professional roles we remain human beings with our own needs for understanding, meaning and purpose. We too struggle to understand what life is about, to answer unanswerable metaphysical questions, to connect with other people and to reach out to transcendent values such as love or beauty. These unanswerable questions undermine our tidy professional barriers to create a personal challenge that may be highly uncomfortable. They force health care professionals to recognise that, for all our professional expertise, we are not experts at being human. Spirituality is a great leveller in health care and while that may be a relief in some ways, it still raises uncomfortable questions that individuals may find difficult, even intolerable.

My experience of reflecting on spirituality with groups of health care professionals suggests that this process actually helped us recognise and cope with our fallibility rather than just make us more aware of it. Once we had overcome our initial difficulties, there was much that was enlightening in exploring spirituality together. These opportunities provided a setting where we could consider difficult questions and issues in a helpful and supportive way, not without its challenges, certainly, but providing a place of mutual support as we recognised our own limitations and vulnerability. Talking about spirituality helped us rediscover what we were about both personally and professionally. Exploring such thorny issues together helped us understand each other better, creating a shared bond that affected our work in many different and beneficial ways. The groups provided an opportunity to tell our own story in a form that integrated spirituality rather than ignoring it and this not only helped us connect with each other but understand and, in time, facilitate such a process with clients. We became more comfortable with our questions and no longer felt we had to have all the answers to other people's questions. Discussions about spirituality provided a framework where we could talk honestly about things we found difficult to understand. The group was not only a place of struggle or disagreement, we were also aware of talking to each other about positive experiences of hope and joy. As such it offered an opportunity for self-care in addition to its important role in developing our service to clients; there was a recognition that this personal exploration of spirituality had benefits for our own health, even our sanity.

A shared understanding of spirituality can no longer be assumed, yet it appears essential for health care teams who wish to work holistically. Continuing professional development provides a forum in which health care staff can specifically explore spirituality and spiritual care in relation to their workplace. Such an exploration is far from being the luxury some might consider it; rather it is the key to developing and embedding an effective holistic care that will benefit both staff and clients. This change of outlook will not be achieved by a short impersonal discussion of the meaning of spirituality – a more complex deliberation that encompasses personal and professional concerns is needed. This in turn requires an appropriate setting where people feel safe to share their personal beliefs and values while they struggle to express their ideas and admit their misunderstandings. Opportunities for health care teams to explore spirituality together in this way provide a useful springboard from which to develop a shared approach to spirituality and spiritual care. An experiential educational approach facilitates an exploration of spirituality and spiritual care that offers both a theoretical overview and an opportunity for more personal reflection. This approach not only increases awareness and understanding of spirituality but enables personal beliefs and values that may be hindering spiritual care provision to be challenged. If such an exploration is to occur and be helpful, there needs to be an understanding both of the issues involved and the group context in which it will occur. This context will be considered in the next chapter.

4

Developing Opportunities to Talk about Spirituality

There is never going to be a quick and easy way to integrate spirituality into the whole of health care. There is a lot to do even for well-established health care teams: starting with the acceptance of spirituality as an issue involving the whole team; moving towards an understanding of spirituality that affects everyone and plays a significant part in health and well-being; recognising how spirituality affects health care professionals personally as well as professionally; considering how practice should respond to this understanding. Opportunities for health care professionals to reflect together about spirituality, drawing on personal and professional experience as well as theoretical ideas, have the potential to make a significant contribution to this process. Teams may choose to do this in differing ways but an understanding of adult learning, including reflective practice, will help ensure that such opportunities affect actual practice in a fruitful and positive way. Time spent exploring spirituality should be a core activity for multi-professional teams aiming to work holistically; if it feels difficult to justify protected time for this (and it will!), perhaps the implications of the commitment to holistic care need to be reconsidered. Other tasks that seem more urgent, and absorb significant amounts of time, may ultimately be less important for actual patient care. We recognise the importance of regular updating on technical aspects of care – the adoption of a similar approach to exploring spirituality in holistic care is no less essential. Health care organisation and management need to support this approach, as do individual clinical staff members.

Offering a group dimension for reflective practice generates a broader spectrum of ideas and opinions – more challenging certainly but also more supportive and resourceful. Groups of individuals bring a range of experiences and ideas about spirituality, creating a wider and deeper picture than is possible for a single individual. Group activity develops its own synergy, enabling the group to achieve things that a single individual is unlikely to achieve alone. Individuals need to overcome their difficulty in speaking openly about spirituality in a public context in order to learn more in this way. Difficult, even painful, issues may be raised during group discussions that challenge comfortable thoughts and beliefs. Hence any group aiming to learn about spirituality must first establish a context where participants are safe to discuss their personal experiences and ideas. That is not to say an easy and over-comfortable space but rather one where it is possible to challenge and be challenged with respect, knowing there is support and understanding when those challenges are uncomfortable. Such discussions may raise difficult issues that spill over into other aspects of the team's work and lead to tension for the whole team. In the same way, external influences, such as individuals who are powerful members of the team in another context, may affect learning as they create barriers that block or limit learning. Practical issues such as physical space and protected time are also important. For all these reasons, a group aiming to learn about spirituality must be established in a way that reduces the risk of problems and enhances the benefits to the team.

Learning continually

If health care teams are to learn about spirituality in this way the approach and context of that learning needs to be considered as carefully as the content. A reflective, experiential approach encourages the integration of theory with practice, while the opportunity to learn with others offers challenge and support. Experienced health care professionals may struggle with this topic, especially if they are less familiar with both the use of personal reflection and a broader view of spirituality. They may come to training sessions expecting, even hoping, that an expert will provide the answers to this difficult subject; they are also likely to experience even greater feelings of anxiety about their own lack of understanding and articulacy. These factors make it particularly important that the ethos and environment of the group are planned and developed carefully in a way that includes all group members.

Creating a safe space in which to explore spirituality is far more than a matter of physical space, yet such practical concerns do have an impact. Learning groups need to meet in a place with adequate space and comfortable seats, where they know they will not be interrupted. It will encourage participation if people know they will not be overheard by non-group members. A room slightly away from the normal working environment may help people relax and 'switch off' without imposing additional demands on time and transport. We were fortunate to have a comfortable shared education room, just outside the normal working environment, that was relatively private and in which the risk of interruptions could be minimised. In a busy clinical area it may help to go elsewhere to meet, even if that is only a short distance away.

Working with groups

A number of basic principles for working with groups, such as respect and a concern for equity, are essential when facilitating discussions about spirituality. It is already clear that this is a sensitive area where the material is essentially exploratory and participants are struggling to express complex ideas that are difficult to articulate. From the very beginning a group dynamic needs to be established that will create an environment in which participants are open to explore, and feel safe to challenge, both their own ideas and those of other people. In order to do this people need to be able to share their experiences, even if they are not sure whether they are relevant or are struggling to put them into words. Where group members hold similar views or express a similar level of uncertainty, discussions may be easier, although possibly less fruitful in the end. Groups that express highly divergent ideas about spirituality, perhaps stemming from the strongly held beliefs of individual members, may find this difficult, particularly if discussions become polarised. The group will need to find ways of recognising and coping with this range of views otherwise individual members may withdraw, either ceasing to be involved in discussions or physically dropping out of the group. Maintaining ground rules such as mutual respect is essential, as is encouraging the group members to listen to each other and look beyond superficial differences. The role of the facilitator is vital to help the group keep to its own ground rules so that participants feel safe and supported. As their confidence grows, they will be more able to express their own tentative ideas about spirituality and something of the struggle involved in this process. Where whole teams of staff are learning together this shared struggle can be an important part of their journey towards mutual understanding, helping them develop and own a consistent approach to spiritual care.

The size of any group exploring spirituality should be sufficiently large to provide enough ideas and resources without reducing participation and discussion, ideally around eight to twelve people. This again raises questions about who should be included; the multi-professional team itself may be larger than this and it is rarely practical for the whole team to be involved at any one time. Not everyone will want to explore spirituality in the same way or to the same extent, as we have already made clear; however, restricting the group to only those people with particular roles or a few key individuals can lead to a feeling of exclusiveness. Other people then feel sidelined or rejected, something that is particularly unhelpful when considering spirituality. This approach also fails to address those in the wider team, such as support staff or professional staff with only occasional contact. A way also needs to be found to draw in new staff as well as offer some form of continuing opportunity for reflection and support.

With these issues very much in mind, the palliative care centre where I worked agreed to offer the whole team the opportunity to take part in an initial exploration of spirituality. This included core professional members such as nursing staff but also individuals such as allied health professionals, complementary therapists and volunteers who had a more marginal role at the care centre. After an open meeting to explore what this process would involve, eight people elected to meet regularly to explore spirituality together. This group took on the task of exploring spirituality in some depth on behalf of the whole team; they reported back to the team at regular intervals and involved other individuals in periodic discussions of the issues involved (see Figure 4.1). One important outcome of this initial exploration was to establish an opportunity for other team members to learn more about what this group had been discovering. Although shorter, these learning opportunities consciously took a very exploratory approach so that participants not only heard what we had learned but were encouraged to discover more for themselves through discussion and personal reflection. Most staff working at the care centre were able to take part in these learning opportunities, including new staff who had joined the centre after the initial project began. These opportunities have continued, with some revisions, and now welcome people from other teams in the area. Details of how to obtain information about the current course are given in Appendix 1. This pattern appeared to balance

Introductory meeting
Brainstorm ideas about spirituality and religion, discuss the format of the group

1st reflection phase
Weekly one-hour sessions for 6 weeks
Agree ground rules and focus of group. Initial focus is on the nature of spirituality. Set first tasks for action period at end of this period

1st action phase
6 weeks
Work individually on agreed tasks that focus on reflection about the nature of personal spirituality

Interim report to centre team

2nd reflection phase
Weekly one-hour sessions for two weeks
Review of action period and agree new tasks as the focus of discussions begins to shift to spiritual care and links with work

2nd action phase
10 weeks
Work individually and in smaller groups on:
- finding out how other centres provide spiritual care
- looking at spiritual assessment questions used by other people

3rd reflection phase
Weekly one hour sessions for 6 weeks
Focus on spiritual care roles, training, being and doing, raising the issue of spirituality with clients

3rd action phase
24 weeks
Work individually and in smaller groups on:
- incorporating spiritual care questions into generic assessment
- developing an educational module about spirituality
- data analysis (facilitator)

Final reflection phase
One two-hour session
Review progress and clarify outcomes for final report

Final report to centre team

Figure 4.1 An outline of the co-operative inquiry process

practical issues with the need to involve the whole team, providing a clear foundation that people could take further if and when they wished.

There is widespread agreement that groups of individuals move through more or less predictable phases of development, which include forming, storming, norming, performing and, sometimes, ending (Tuckman 1965). A collection of slightly subdued individuals start by 'forming' themselves into a group; they move into 'storming' mode as those individuals begin to speak out and challenge each other in ways that may lead to conflict or tension; they settle into 'norming' as the group members understand and work within their own established rules and patterns of activity; and finally reach the 'performing' stage where the group has a life of its own and is getting down to the task in hand in a beneficial and concerted way. Most groups will end, formally or informally, as individuals leave or the task is completed. There may be a reluctance to reach this final stage even when their task is complete because of the loss of support and friendship as well as the sense of achievement and purpose linked to the task itself. Of course, an established multi-professional team should already be 'performing', although this new topic is likely to call for a rather different approach that may unsettle the group, disturbing normal roles and patterns of behaviour. Re-establishing and maintaining performance will not happen without a great deal of work on the part of all the group members. This work may be quite personal as individuals reflect on their own beliefs and experiences in the light of what they are learning through the group. It may also be more outward-looking as people consciously, sometimes with difficulty, listen to the different perspectives provided by other group members or theoretical material being considered.

Although the overall focus on spirituality was agreed, the groups I worked with chose a democratic style where the whole group was involved in agreeing an aim and approach, including ground rules. In the longer-running open discussion group, individual members brought their own topics for discussion throughout rather than having a pre-arranged plan, although as facilitator I did bring some materials to help get discussion started until the group began to discover its own resources and ideas. The learning groups for other staff that met later had, of necessity, a shorter time span and a more specific educational purpose. This helped some staff to take part more easily but meant that an outline syllabus needed to be agreed in advance to ensure best use of limited time. Within this overall plan, there was still a strong emphasis on group members contributing to discussions and bringing examples and ideas from their own experience. All the groups I worked with exhibited these differing stages of group life, whether or not they were already part of a well-established team. It was as if we needed to get to know each other in a different way when we began to talk about spirituality – something that was not normally discussed openly. In the longest-running group a significant part of the early sessions was spent reflecting on the nature of spirituality. We needed to formulate our own ideas about spirituality, testing assumptions and preconceptions against the new information gleaned from theoretical information and from each other. I suspect this time was also part of forming the group, as we needed to listen to each other and develop an increased sense of trust as we began to discuss an area that was new and personal. For myself, involved in a number of different groups, this first stage provided space to tease out the varied ideas and experiences of people in the group from which shared themes gradually emerged. For another individual, a key moment was the recognition that belief in a human spiritual dimension did not conflict with a humanistic viewpoint. Again, for one group, a pivotal experience was recognising and agreeing that spirituality is an innate potential in each human being that may be expressed in different ways.

Such key moments of recognition can precipitate a shift in thinking or approach. For example, in the group just referred to there was a significant sense of moving on from highly personal discussions to more practical issues about spiritual care after this recognition. In this group several individuals returned after a short break from regular meetings to report significant personal developments in their understanding of spirituality, as though the break offered time to absorb what they had been learning, giving them a chance to reflect and clarify their thinking; the whole group was then able to consider more work-related issues with a renewed sense of purpose. The reflective group approach requires individual group members to recognise and accept their own part in learning; rather than a passive acceptance of information this is an active commitment to learning together. This approach, which may be unfamiliar to some group members, is certainly not an easy process but I would suggest that it brings its own rewards.

The role of the facilitator

Where groups are meeting to learn about spirituality, it is often helpful to appoint an agreed facilitator, someone who can help the group agree and meet its learning aims as well as support practical and organisational issues. This could be someone outside the group who is given the specific task of facilitation or it could be a role adopted by different individuals within the group for a period of time. In established multi-professional teams it will be important to discuss the issue of facilitation openly and reach agreement about who will facilitate the group. An individual who leads the group in another sphere may not be the best person to facilitate discussions about spirituality; for example, the power they wield within that other context may make it difficult for other group members to contribute freely in discussions. Equally, if learning is to be experienced by the whole group, someone perceived as an expert in spirituality may not be the best facilitator; individuals who lack confidence about spirituality may defer too easily to someone they view as an expert and be more reluctant to express their own ideas. A facilitator who is seen as neutral by the group, rather than a core member of the team, may be of benefit. Someone with experience and understanding of the process of adult education would be ideally suited to such a role, whether or not they also have an understanding of health care. I certainly found my knowledge of adult and continuing education invaluable in facilitating the learning groups with which I was involved, perhaps even more essential than my own experience in health care. Indeed, someone who is not a health care professional may be more easily able to challenge ideas that are taken for granted by the multi-professional team. It is essential that the approach to facilitation is discussed at an early stage, and agreement reached by the whole group to avoid tension and difficulty later.

The facilitator requires the group's support in order to fulfil a demanding role; he or she is part of the group yet remains slightly on its margins in order to support the development and life of the group. The facilitator needs the support of the whole group in ensuring that ground rules are adhered to and learning occurs, but equally the group members will need the facilitator to remind them of what has been agreed and to help them avoid getting diverted from their main purpose. By their very nature, discussions about spirituality tend to roam far and wide as people push at the boundaries of what they think spirituality is. This is a valuable part of the process and needs to be encouraged but it can mean that groups lose sight of their agreed aim. The groups I worked with had the clearly agreed aim 'to explore our own spirituality with a view to how that informs our work'. We needed to be reminded of that aim when we took each other down interesting byways and theoretical dead ends. Initially some rambling was expected as people tentatively approached questions about each other's beliefs or experience; we needed that space as we learned to trust each other. Later our discussions became more focused as the group began to perform at its agreed task of exploring spirituality specifically in relation to our work and then diversions became less helpful. Spirituality, by its very nature, did seem to raise endlessly fascinating topics for conversation and I suspect some members of the group were enjoying a rare opportunity for philosophical exploration.

The facilitator plays an important practical role in the organisation of the group, ensuring that meeting times are agreed, rooms booked, information disseminated, even if some of this activity is shared or delegated within the group. The facilitator can initiate and lead the group's discussions, particularly in the early sessions, but should always encourage group participation rather than imposing his or her own views. Perhaps more importantly the facilitator plays a vital role in managing the life of the group, using his or her skills to ensure that the group's aim is first agreed and then achieved. This may proceed smoothly with little intervention from the facilitator but my experience is that it often does not. Agreeing and achieving its aims requires the whole group to become a resource for learning, with all participants feeling that they can and should contribute to discussions. The facilitator may need to challenge apparent assumptions on behalf of the group, encourage and motivate quieter members to contribute and ensure that ground rules are not only agreed but maintained. The group's help can be enlisted in all these processes but someone needs to make sure that they happen. I certainly found it demanding to facilitate the groups I was involved in. Aiming to model an open approach to learning about spirituality, I made it clear that I did not have all the answers but I still needed to resist pressure to act as an expert on occasion. Interestingly, neither myself nor the co-facilitator involved in the educational groups was a chaplain, although both of us had additional experience of pastoral care and of teaching about spirituality. Shared facilitation helped model a multi-professional approach to spiritual care, particularly as we were from different professional groups and worked in different areas of the organisation. As co-facilitators, we found it essential to meet regularly to reflect on how the group was developing, to review the content and explore our own involvement. We also needed to be aware of our own spirituality and the impact it had on our work, including our involvement with the educational groups, and it was helpful to reflect on this together. We worked hard to remain open to new ways of thinking that emerged within the group rather than attempting to impose, even unconsciously, our own views; our role was not to talk too much ourselves but rather to draw out other members of the group.

An important dilemma for facilitators is how open to be about their own beliefs and values; education about spirituality cannot realistically be value-free even when not aiming to impose a particular viewpoint. It seemed incongruous to shut away my own ideas about spirituality, but equally I did not want those ideas to be a barrier to others. Part of my personal work as facilitator within the different groups with which I worked was to recognise my own agenda in terms of spirituality, trying to ensure that this was also open to exploration by the group. I frequently found myself challenged by our discussions and recognised that my own ideas changed and developed over time.

Clear discussions about ground rules, particularly those ensuring respect for individual beliefs, are vitally important from the earliest stage of any group. Ground rules should be discussed openly and agreed within the team, but that is only the beginning. It is also important that they are adhered to and the facilitator, as well as the group itself, plays a pivotal role in this. The ground rules established by the groups with which I was involved all included statements about confidentiality and mutual respect.

All the groups expressed their concern to get the right balance between encouraging the whole group to participate and refusing to pressurise people to contribute where they felt unable or unwilling to do so. All group members were eager to learn together but understood this would be challenging, and were particularly conscious of the need to be sensitive about deeply held personal beliefs. People in the group that met to explore spirituality for longest placed the greatest emphasis on the responsibility of each individual to contribute and take part in discussions. Perhaps these self-selected individuals were already highly motivated to learn about this area and felt an additional responsibility to explore on behalf of the wider team. In practice, all the groups experienced stormy patches as they explored together and there were often challenging sessions. Some individuals inevitably contributed more than others but everyone did take part, with quieter members often playing a valuable role as they reflected on ideas that had been skimmed over by more voluble members of the group.

One particular point of tension in all the groups was the difference between exploring and arriving, pointing to the wider tension, already discussed, to do with having or not having answers. There was a general acceptance within the groups that spirituality is a lifelong process of exploration, again often linked to the idea of the journey. Some individuals were conscious that this sense of exploration was integral to their own thinking about spirituality; others were equally clear that they had arrived at a place where they felt they belonged and further exploration would only be from this more settled base. This tension affected the group activity, with some individuals clearly wanting the whole group to arrive at a particular point and others resisting this pressure:

I'm just so fixed on the journey that to me the questions are what interests me. As soon as someone says they've arrived I feel they've found something I'm excluded from. I can never be there because for me it's the journey and it will always be the journey. That's where my spirituality lies.

This important difference reflected personalities as well as values and beliefs and is likely to be significant in any group discussing spirituality. Our groups needed to recognise the tension and respond to it rather than allow it to fester or hinder performance outside the group.

Adults learning

All those involved in learning about spirituality in health care will be adults. Such adult learners bring a wealth of experience and insight, both positive and negative, to any learning experience; they also tend to be more ready to learn where they feel the subject is directly relevant to their role or will help resolve problems they actually experience. This can be a great advantage when spirituality is understood to play a significant role in holistic care, although some explanation may be needed to help people see its relevance. A less positive aspect is that misunderstandings about spirituality may have a negative effect on motivation and learning; the tacit belief that spirituality is really all about religion, for example, may encourage some health care staff to attend but others to stay away, as well as causing tension within the learning group. Adult health care professionals may arrive expecting to be given the answers to their questions about spirituality and be resistant to a more experiential approach that seems to have few answers and makes them work to find out more. Such expectations are changing as reflection is used increasingly in both initial and post-registration health care training. However, it is still important that participants are able to reflect at an early stage on the relevance of spirituality to their own practice and the reasons for choosing a reflective experiential style.

Although I am suggesting that multi-professional health care teams provide an ideal setting in which to learn about spirituality, it is not possible (or indeed ethical) to force people to learn about it in this way. Some persuasion, or at least initial explanation, may be needed to encourage people to become involved in educational groups about spirituality; otherwise self-selection of those who are already interested will hinder the involvement of the whole team in this area of care. Short introductory sessions, perhaps a day course or introductory lunchtime update, may help break down misconceptions about spirituality so that individual staff sense its relevance to their work and perhaps feel less threatened by these ideas. New staff may be introduced to these ideas through induction or mentoring, perhaps reflecting on spiritual aspects of critical incidents or particular case studies. Clinical supervision, now becoming established within health care, is another opportunity where spiritual concerns may safely be explored, although this relies on those who provide supervision being familiar with the concepts involved. Despite the growing interest in some areas of health care, I sense there is still a widespread failure to understand the relevance of spirituality to the wider health care community, although this may change as the factors discussed earlier take effect.

Using relevant experience in their learning is important as a way of motivating adults and may encourage more personal and individual reflection. If all health care staff are encouraged to practise holistically, they need to understand what this means in theory and practice, and that should include understanding spirituality. Continuing professional education should encourage this learning to complement more technical and practical aspects of health care. If it becomes more widely accepted that there is a need for health care staff to learn about spirituality, then it also becomes important to think how best such learning can be achieved. A short lecture within a formal course may, helpfully, highlight the issues involved but the opportunity to develop the sort of shared understanding that influences personal and professional practice needs a rather different approach. What is needed is an approach that will allow health care professionals to both increase their awareness of the issues involved and develop greater confidence about their ability, thus helping to overcome the significant theory–practice gap existing in this area. Particular moments in professional development can be used as a catalyst to encourage staff to learn about spirituality. These might include coping with death or serious illness, or being present at a birth. Such experiences can be explored within clinical supervision or informally with peers and more experienced staff. However, educational opportunities like the ones I have described provide an additional opportunity to explore such experiences in a wider context. An experiential approach to learning assists that process by specifically encouraging participants to explore spirituality in relation to their own personal and professional experience. The degree of personal challenge this involves may be uncomfortable and the potential difficulties of working with experience for participants and tutors should not be underestimated. A purely theoretical stance may even be adopted by participants in order to distance themselves when the content becomes too challenging. The cultural bias towards cognitive and skills-based education within health care adds to the difficulties of learning about spirituality. Previous educational experiences that emphasised knowledge or skills in isolation from experience create a barrier for some health care professionals who do not recognise this more experiential approach as valid learning, particularly when it involves such a personal subject!

In fact, a significant proportion of the people I worked with described the way in which their own personal experiences, at home and at work, were what motivated them to explore spiritual issues. It was for this reason that the overall aim of groups I worked with was to develop a richer and more grounded understanding of spirituality. This enabled us to draw on a wide range of ideas and experiences, our own and those of other people, as well as more theoretical written material. In this way we did not just learn isolated theory but an understanding of spirituality that became internalised, affecting our lives and work. Personal exploration was clearly an essential part of our learning but our primary focus was not personal spiritual development for its own sake. Our aim was to develop an understanding of spirituality that would both be informed by and inform our working practice. The groups I worked with all had a sense of people sharing their stories with each other – personal disclosure that can leave individuals vulnerable but also offers an opportunity to see things differently, to find new ways of understanding and interpreting our own experience in the light of what we can learn from each other.

Opportunities to learn about spirituality need to include time for people to tell their own stories. Stories are more than simple remembrance; both storyteller and listener reflect their sense of what is important, gaining an opportunity to organise and shape their experience, to gain new insight. People tell stories to organise and shape their experience and this sense of a personal narrative can be an important coping strategy in illness (Burton 1998). For example, someone reflected on the way in which a discussion with a client about eating and weight loss brought greater insight into changing roles within his home and family life, leading to better understanding of his own loss of identity and fear about the future. Another person talked about the experience of looking through old photographs and how it connected with her changing understanding of spirituality, making her think more about who people really are and what remains of that essential human being as people change and grow old or ill.

Discussions like this kept us grounded, prompting us to consider how our own spirituality was related to everyday activities and roles as well as philosophical ideas. Sharing this exploration with each other helped us to recognise and respect the same process when it occurred with patients and carers; we noticed afresh how the stories we had heard from patients influenced the way we worked. The examples we shared with other people, the way we heard what clients were saying, how we treated other clients were all shaped by our experiences. Integrating those experiences into our learning gave us time to look beyond the superficial facts of an experience and helped create a sense of connection within the group.

Participants need to be clear about the commitment they are entering into and time constraints should be agreed and respected. It may help if the meetings have a clear pattern that includes time to gather together, a recognised opening and ending, in addition to the central educational and reflective activity. The timing of our sessions varied but most occurred at the end of the working day as the care centre was closing, enabling participants to use a mixture of their own time and work time. In two of the groups, refreshments were available as people arrived. This both supported those who had travelled some distance and created a break between work and learning group. Each session began with a period of open reflection; making this apparent from the first session helped participants contribute as they were able to come prepared. Communication both before and during the group needed to be clear, helping individuals to be involved by ensuring they understood what was happening even if they had missed a session. As facilitator of one long-running group, I produced brief notes immediately after each session and these were circulated to the group for comment and communication. This helped include anyone who had missed a session but also provided a record of our discussions and a starting point for the following session. Similarly the educational groups that I co-facilitated had a pre-arranged outline programme, including dates and topics, that participants were given in advance. (Appendix 2 includes suggestions for groups to consider when exploring spirituality; Appendix 1 explains where to obtain details of the current course.)

Working with reflection

Reflective practice is now well established as a method in the education of health care professionals, offering a grounded process that values both human experience and theoretical concepts. Reflection offers an opportunity to develop knowledge that connects with the real issues of professional practice, trying to work out what new understandings mean in the confines of work and organisational structures. Schon's work is often quoted, including the following metaphor for professional development:

> In the varied topography of professional practice, there is a high, hard ground overlooking a swamp. On the high ground, manageable problems lend themselves to solution through the application of research based theory and technique. In the swampy lowlands, messy confusing problems defy technical solution. The irony of this situation is that the problems of the high ground tend to be relatively unimportant to individuals or society at large...while in the swamp lie the problems of greatest human concern. (Schon 1988, p.3)

Learning usefully about spirituality is definitely swamp-based! In reality most learning involves attitudes and emotions as well as thinking and practical skills. Reflection on and in experience ensures theory is tested out against reality with the specific aim of bridging the gap between theory and practice, something particularly relevant to spirituality, as discussed in earlier chapters. The direct concerns and questions raised by working practice provide both a place to start and a point of reference for learning. Ideas generated by a theoretical exploration are illuminated by experience, which in turn generates more ideas. Of course, as we have already discussed, group reflection needs to occur in an environment that will both challenge and support participants, particularly when it involves issues that are difficult to articulate and emotionally challenging. Familiar ideas become comfortable, so that it is difficult to see other ways of doing things. When assumptions are recognised, the effect of these ideas on practice becomes more transparent and open, so that reflection may lead to change or affirmation.

The groups that I worked with experienced a cycle of learning as we consciously reflected on our experience, relating that learning to the growing body of literature we were discovering and in turn measuring that literature against our own experience. In this process our confidence and understanding of the topic grew, particularly as our discussions, although based within health care, were also open to ideas from the media and the Arts, from religious and non-religious groups and other areas of our experience and background. This fuelled a broader discussion that was particularly relevant to a topic like spirituality and I was interested to read theatre critic Michael Billington's suggestion that the Arts are what now remind people of spiritual questions:

> Even a supposedly secular society retains its hunger for mystery, with art now fulfilling the function once exercised by divine service. It satisfies our need for the numinous...theatre, music and visual art are what really stir our spiritual longings. (Billington 1999, p.4)

I am not trying to suggest that we set up groups to discuss our ideas about art and theatre but rather that we remain open to insights from outside health care. Specific opportunities to reflect on experience were built into all the learning; groups and individuals were encouraged to continue reflection between sessions, using a reflective diary where possible. Such a journal provides a powerful tool for professional development as it 'taps the unconscious, it can make the implicit explicit and therefore open to inquiry' (Holly 1989, p.71). Time to reflect together was included in all group discussions although diaries remained personal and private to each individual. In the longest-running inquiry group, there was a deliberate pattern of alternating periods of reflection and action both between weekly sessions and over longer periods. In the shorter educational groups, in the first week participants were encouraged to start their reflective journal during the session. Everyone was encouraged to take the difficult first step of writing something down, so that it would be easier to continue this written reflection process. All subsequent sessions of the group began with a period of open sharing, drawing on reflective diaries where appropriate; there was also a bulletin board available for people to bring stories, articles, poems or press cuttings they had discovered; this was well used. In the specific educational groups, with a more established syllabus, we were conscious of the risk that theoretical content would squeeze out opportunities to reflect on personal experience and we worked hard to resist this temptation.

Creativity, symbol, story, metaphor and ritual all offer different ways of talking about spirituality and these different approaches were used in all the groups, even when they felt strange and unfamiliar. For example, the journey was a recurring theme in our discussions but specifically discussing other metaphors for spirituality drew out alternative images such as weaving, different types of garden, and light and darkness, and suggested themes such as growth, energy, connectedness and depth. The purpose of metaphors is said to be to 'express the inexpressible' (Candy 1986) and they should be considered particularly useful when referring to spirituality. An opportunity to discuss metaphors for spirituality confirmed the distinctiveness of ideas about spirituality as participants recognised how strongly some individuals felt about particular images. At the end of each short course every participant had the opportunity to talk briefly to the whole group about an article (such as a book or picture) they felt spoke strongly about their own spirituality. This seemed to provide an important opportunity for individuals to draw together what they had learnt and sometimes express their spirituality in a new way.

A commitment to spirituality as continuing professional development

Commitment to continuing professional development is a basic requirement for most health care staff, important for maintaining competency to practise as well as for learning about new skills or techniques (Department of Health 1998, pp.41–9). The Knowledge and Skills Framework for the National Health Service (Department of Health 2004b) describes the essential knowledge and skills that NHS staff require for their work. Communication, personal development, and equality and diversity – areas that underpin holistic care – are core dimensions required by all staff. More specific dimensions, required by some groups of staff, recognise health and well-being as encompassing emotional, mental, physical, social and spiritual needs. Staff are required to provide evidence demonstrating that they meet these dimensions at differing levels depending on the detailed requirements of their job. Taking part in a multi-professional team exploration of spirituality, and reflecting how this has influenced personal and professional development, would be one way of demonstrating that this dimension is being met. Another way would be to use the experience of the group to reflect on the holistic care of a particular client, perhaps showing the integration of spiritual care with other health needs.

This growing emphasis on evidence for clinical outcomes and effective practice is closely linked with current ideas about continuing professional development within the National Health Service (Department of Health 1998, pp.33–8). This trend, combined with the initiatives outlined in Chapter 2, should encourage opportunities for continuing professional development about spirituality, but sadly this does not yet appear to be the case in pre or post education about health. Interestingly, an international work group on death, dying and bereavement (Spiritual Care Work Group 1990) also noted the need for continuing spiritual education within health care; its list of the assumptions and principles of spiritual palliative care deserves to be more widely discussed. Other writers have also highlighted the need for effective education to prepare staff to recognise and respond to spirituality in their clients (for example, Narayanasamy 1991; Harrison and Burnard 1993; Bradshaw 1994; Ross 1998; Smith 1999; McSherry 2000). Health care chaplains are sometimes, unreasonably, expected to have all the skills required in this area and also recognise the need to develop practical competence in this area through continuing professional development (Kerry 2001).

While the importance of including spirituality in the education of health care staff is becoming more recognised, there is still uncertainty about how this should be done. It is clear that spirituality touches on deeply personal issues as well as professional concerns and there is a natural concern about taking the right approach. The gap between theory and practice we have already noted implies that an effective approach to teaching spirituality has not yet been found. Bradshaw (1994) highlights the risks of simply bolting something onto an already full nursing curriculum and suggests that spirituality should be 'caught' by example and experience rather than formally taught. Yet the opposite may occur; in a world where spirituality is already neglected and confused, no learning will occur because there is little spontaneous discussion of spirituality and few visible examples of spiritual care in action. Indeed, the real danger is that health care professionals will actually learn to avoid this area or acquire unhelpful skills that will lead to further neglect.

Using reflection on and in experience as an approach to learning about spirituality, as I have been describing, seems to offer a helpful way forward in education about spirituality. There is now far more recognition of the benefits of reflection and experiential learning and a greater emphasis on outcomes in health care education and practice. Spirituality remains a difficult topic to learn about for all the reasons already discussed. It is sometimes easier to stick to topics that are more easily explained and assessed, but this will not bring about the changes required. What is needed in learning about spirituality is not necessarily new knowledge or new initiatives but rather the opportunity to implement what is already known more widely and in practical ways. Reflecting on a survey of spirituality among Belgian palliative care staff, Cornette seems to sum this up:

> The first thing to do, therefore, in order to optimise actual spiritual care given is not to develop new projects that deal with spiritual pain on a more theoretical level. Help must first be given to palliative care teams themselves to implement their knowledge in their daily work. If this implementation is to be done seriously, regular supervision, either individually or on a team basis, where care givers can look in safety at their personal spiritual agenda, is a pre-requisite. (1997, p.13)

There is a great need for personal learning about spirituality to be related to more formal continuing professional development frameworks at all levels of health care study and for all professions. Opportunities for continuing professional education about spirituality in health care settings, rather than academia, are particularly important. Spirituality should be essential knowledge for all health care practitioners who work directly with clients as is implied, to a limited degree, within the NHS Knowledge and Skills Framework (Department of Health 2004b).

As we have seen, spirituality cannot be simply taught in the same way as a practical skill or theoretical idea but opportunities to explore and reflect can nurture spirituality given time and encouragement. This process affects the individuals who take part but also the teams and organisations to which they belong. Learning about spirituality in health care, even where that learning includes reflection on experience, should never comprise the whole of an individual's personal spiritual development. However, it does provide a valuable addition to other activities that nurture the spirit; for some people it may start the process of exploring their own spirituality in other ways. These could include a whole range of creative pursuits such as writing, arts and crafts or music as well as gardening or cooking, or meditation, being in the countryside or in contact with nature. Greater awareness of spirituality, its nature and concerns, supports a more balanced and discerning holistic approach that engenders a sense of well-being and has very direct practical outcomes, as these two participants have realised:

> The course encouraged me to think much more deeply about the real concerns of people in a practical way.

> It's about creating opportunities to address spiritual needs, and being aware not to close down dialogue through our own fears or lack of understanding.

So, having recognised the need to learn about spirituality and considered how this can be done in group settings, we move on to reflect on the nature of spirituality itself. Although spirituality is commonly linked to religion, as I have already intimated, it should be considered in a much broader, more inclusive way. This understanding is particularly important when considering spirituality, which is relevant to all those, clients and health care staff, involved in health care. Recognising spirituality as a unique potential within each person, as we shall do in the following chapters, opens new possibilities for considering its place within holistic care. It also provides the starting point for a view of spiritual care that pertains to everyone.

5

Understanding Spirituality

Spirituality is an idea that appears to resonate with our postmodern western world-view. Searching the Internet, surely a symbol of modern life, shows thousands of sites related to spirituality. Referred to in many different contexts, it is frequently linked to such diverse subjects as gardening, the environment, the Arts, sport, lifestyle, even shopping. Yet the essence of spirituality remains elusive and underlying this genuine interest there appears to be little clarity about the nature of spirituality. This lack of understanding leaves individuals ill equipped to discern what is of lasting value in all this talk of spirituality, to recognise when this popular phrase is simply being used as a marketing ploy. In health care in particular, this failure to understand spirituality hinders attempts to work holistically and may leave individuals vulnerable to misunderstanding and even duplicity. Although it appears impossible to reach a consensus where there are such widely differing views, a number of themes echo through most discussions about spirituality. The link between human spirituality and existential questions about meaning and purpose seems to be at the heart of these themes. Multi-professional teams wishing to explore spirituality would find it helpful to consider spirituality and related themes in relationship to their area of work.

A foundation for understanding

Traditionally the word 'spirit' or 'soul' is linked to the breath or the animating principle of life, a link seen in words such as inspire and inspiration. The *Shorter Oxford English Dictionary* (Little *et al.* 1973) defines 'spirit' in this sense as:

> The animating or vital principal in man and animals; that which gives life to the physical organism, in contrast to its purely material elements; the breath of life.

Hence, spirituality can be understood as the essence of each human being, distinctive yet inseparable from the physical and intellectual. As such it is an aspect of life that is vital and yet so much a part of everyday experience that it is easily overlooked. Other definitions add to this sense that the spiritual is both other-worldly and essential. Looking at a dictionary again suggests other interesting links: for example, 'spirit' can refer to supernatural beings or ghosts as well as to distilled volatile liquids such as alcohol (Little *et al.* 1973). Indeed, *l'eau de vie* (water of life), the French phrase for distilled spirit, highlights this particular link! A related understanding links spirituality to elements of everyday life, such as beauty or love, that transcend the physical and material as they reach towards the ultimate or eternal. I particularly like the deceptively straightforward description of spirituality as 'human concern for the things that matter' (Whipp 1998, p.139), although I suspect there would be a lot to learn in unpacking what that actually means.

Discernible within some of these ideas about spirituality is a sense of the separation or otherness of the spiritual from the body and mind. Perhaps this reflects the culture from which they emerge but this is in direct contrast to the more holistic understanding that body, mind and spirit are integrated in the whole being. If the human spirit is distinct yet inseparable from body and mind then spiritual concerns can be expressed only through physical and mental processes; the spiritual can be neglected but there is a cost to the body and mind. Conversely, where the spiritual is nurtured there are benefits to mind and body. Returning to the idea of breath reminds us that human beings are an integrated whole; the very physical action of breathing (inspiration) shows body, mind and spirit working in intricate, unconscious harmony. This physical activity both enables and influences the whole. Thoughts and feelings influence the muscles and nerves that in turn affect our breathing, as anyone will understand who has experienced the changes in breathing brought about by stress or relaxation.

Mind and body work together even though we are often unaware of the links, but what about the spirit? Perhaps we are even less aware of the link between breathing and the human spirit but what about the sharp intake of breath at an unexpectedly glorious scene or a deepening of our breathing when meditating? Indeed, how could we ever appreciate beauty or experience love without that essential act of breathing? Ceasing to breathe still marks a significant end to any life, body, mind or spirit.

Underpinning ideas

If, then, spirituality is accepted as an integral element of each person, there remains an even more pressing need to understand what that actually means. Spirituality is being discussed more frequently within health care as an element of the holistic approach but its inherent complexity, combined with the difficulty of describing and quantifying it, ensures it remains on the sidelines of actual practice. Developing an understanding of spirituality that works in an organisational context rather than only for individuals is even more difficult:

> Definitions [of spirituality] exist but these may not suit all conditions. The difficulty reflects the struggle – personal and organisational – to encapsulate an intangible essence which for many people gives the truest meaning of them and their lives. (Keighley 1997, p.47)

Members of the exploring spirituality groups that I worked with discussed a number of definitions of spirituality, some of which are given in Box 5.1, but remained reluctant to define spirituality too closely themselves. We preferred to identify key themes and concepts that could be used as a base from which to describe and explore spirituality as outlined in this chapter. This process of exploration relieved our initial confusion and helped members of the group gain confidence about working within this broader understanding of spirituality. As one group member stated:

> I think the more you explore the more you realise how immensely different it is for people and how answers is probably the very wrong end of the spectrum to come from. So it's supporting each other to become more [confident] without the answers. Sometimes, it's when you haven't got answers, that's the time when you do block... So that's the good thing to bring it back into a forum from which we can explore.

Spirituality, we suggested, could be understood broadly as an innate potential within all human beings that was concerned with connection, meaning, hope and other existential concerns. This initially sounded rather remote and

---

Box 5.1 Definitions of spirituality

Those attitudes, beliefs and practices which animate people's lives and help them reach out to super-sensible realities. (Adapted from Wakefield 1983)

The essence inside you that makes you aware that things are not just physical or financial. Something that helps you function as a human being and gives meaning and purpose. (Adapted from Wilmer 1997)

The power within a person's life that gives meaning, purpose and fulfilment; the will to live; the belief in self, in others and in a power beyond self that is centred in God. (Adapted from Renetzky 1979)

A quality that goes beyond religious affiliation; that strives for inspiration, reverence, awe, meaning and purpose, even in those who do not believe in any god. The spiritual dimension tries to be in harmony with the universe, strives for answers about the infinite and comes into focus when the person faces emotional stress, physical illness and death. (Adapted from Murray and Zentner 1988)

---

theoretical but as we talked about what we meant, we began to recognise that such themes were an integral part of many everyday life events for ourselves and our clients: relationships with others, experience of the natural world, art or music, as well as specifically religious or spiritual experiences. Similarly we came to see that spirituality could be expressed and developed in many different ways – for example, through creative activities and relationships as well as religious activity, through a simple delight in life or appreciating the beauty of a particular scene. We were beginning to understand that spirituality could be important whatever people's attitude to religion and that certain events, notably birth, ill health and death, could stimulate a greater interest and awareness about spirituality. Sometimes this interest provoked difficult questions but at other times we also saw how it led to a heightened awareness of the value of life, a sense of wonder or renewed purpose. As people who worked in health care, we became even more aware of how we had been affected by other people's spirituality, including how people responded to illness or lived their lives.

As we explored the concept of spirituality together we found a growing agreement about certain key elements within our understanding. Not that we all agreed with each other about everything, of course, but within our differ-ences we found that a common core was emerging. We understood our own ideas better as well as each other's and some of those ideas seemed less distant than they had initially appeared now that we had explored them together. As one group member explained:

> I know that's what you see and feel and believe. It's not what I see, feel and believe but I do think there is a middle ground of things that we would agree on.

Our individual confidence and awareness of spirituality grew in parallel with this shared understanding and this enabled us to integrate these ideas into our practice both as individuals and as a team. It is these core elements of our understanding (outlined in Box 5.2) that I propose to explore further in this chapter before considering the place of spiritual care in health care practice.

Box 5.2 Key themes to be explored

Spirituality is…

- an innate potential in every person
- unique to each individual
- the essence of being human
- integrated not separated from body and mind
- transcendent but not isolated from everyday experiences
- to be nurtured
- linked to meaning, hope, connection with others
- Not the same as religion, although it might be linked.

Unique, innate potential

First and foremost within our exploratory group came a growing acceptance that spirituality is an innate potential in each and every human being. Echoing earlier suggestions that spirituality is as vital as breathing, this idea is widely recognised in other writing about spirituality in health care. In 1990, the World Health Organization's expert committee on palliative care noted the need for spirituality to be recognised as an essential element of the holistic approach while, in 1996, the National Association of Health Authorities and Trusts argued that 'It seems reasonable to argue that there is, in the widest sense of the word, a potentially spiritual dimension for everyone. This will manifest itself in different ways' (1996, p.6).

This universality is echoed in other guidelines, including those issued by the European LUCAS group (a multidisciplinary group based in Leuven, comprising palliative care staff and pastors/theologians; see Cornette 1997) and the Department of Health (2003a). Recognising spirituality as innate and universal was the first key element that we were able to agree as a group. By 'innate' the group intended to suggest that spirituality was an intrinsic element of simply being human. Returning to definitions, the *Shorter Oxford English Dictionary* (Little *et al.* 1973) implies this when it describes innate as something that is 'possessed at birth'. If spirituality is considered to be innate it is in some way an integral part of our genetic make-up. Benson, the American doctor quoted earlier, describes human beings as 'wired for God' (Benson with Stark 1996, pp.196–8), implying that the instinct for belief, worship or prayer is related to survival. Interestingly, spiritual experiences are common even in today's supposedly secular world, again suggesting that spirituality is a resilient element of human nature (see the summary in Box 5.3). Alastair Hardy, founder of the Religious Experience Research Unit (now known as the Alastair Hardy Research Centre), believed that such awareness is widespread because it plays a role in human survival (Hay 1990, p.23).

Our group certainly did not make such a specific link with human survival and a divine being or religious belief, but adopted the wider idea that spirituality is built into human nature. Although this idea is widely accepted, it assumed a new significance as we began to tease out what that meant for our own lives and working practice. If we really believed spirituality to be innate, then it had to follow that it could be relevant to each individual (client, carer or staff), with all their differences of ideas and understandings. It was relevant even for individuals who had no thought of their own spirituality or who may choose to ignore it. As a potential it could be nurtured and developed and would be expressed in many different ways. We began to see that spirituality needed to be an integral part of our overall service, relevant to staff and clients, however they chose to express this aspect of themselves. Once this foundation was accepted our discussions turned more towards ways in which the potential human spirit could be nurtured and encouraged, accepting that this may happen in many different ways. We accepted that some individuals would choose to ignore the spiritual but increasingly felt that this would be to their detriment and that we would want to encourage people to consider and

Box 5.3 Spiritual experiences

Adverts invited contact from individuals who 'have been conscious of, and perhaps influenced by, some such power, whether they call it God or not, to write a simple and brief account of these feelings and their effects'.

There was a small response from the religious press but a much greater response from a general advert and the Unit recorded approximately 4000 accounts of such experiences by 1980 (Hardy 1979).

Later, the question, 'Have you ever been aware of or influenced by a presence or power, whether you call it God or not, which is different from your everyday self?' was included in a National Opinion Poll survey. The response showed that about 36 per cent of respondents have had such experiences that were often very fleeting, and more likely to occur when people were alone, distressed or in contact with nature. Similar results had been seen in America (35% of respondents) where religious groups were thought to be stronger. Subsequently, a random sample of 100 adults in Nottingham (50 women and 50 men) were interviewed. Over 60 per cent claimed that they had had an experience of this kind, suggesting that people are more likely to talk about intimate experiences in an in-depth interview (Hay 1982, 1990).

develop this area of their lives. The practical effect of this as related to spiritual care will be expanded upon in the next chapter.

A clear, parallel recognition for the group was the sense that spirituality is as unique as any other aspect of our humanity. Perhaps that seems obvious, yet it was profoundly liberating to realise that it was not necessary to be the same as anyone else in order to be a spiritual being:

> If someone talks to me about spirituality and what it is, it's always seemed to me that it's got rules and parameters and this is how it is – 'Oh well you're not very spiritual then.' So I really like that idea. Why should it be the same for anyone else? Why can't it be as unique as everything else about us that's unique? And it doesn't mean you haven't got it.

This felt a very important freedom to individuals within the group, in some cases reflecting previous experience where there had been attempts to impose particular views of spirituality. Rather than impose any specific form of spirituality, we wanted to ensure that individual differences were valued and respected while encouraging an exploration of what was held in common.

Spirituality as essence or core

Agreeing that the spiritual is innate and unique still gives little indication about what the spirit is, although it does suggest that it should not be ignored. A common view of spirituality is that it is the essence or core of what it is to be human. For example, this view can be sensed in Ross's suggestion that the spiritual dimension is 'A central artery, which permeates, energises and enlivens the other dimensions of humankind…around which all values, thoughts, decisions, behaviours, experiences and other concerns revolve' (1997a, p.38). This hints further at links with key themes such as meaning, purpose and connection, which will be explored later, and retains a sense of integration. This idea of essence always carries the risk of implying that the spiritual is somehow independent, even superior, to the body and mind, something we have already been at pains to dispute. Where the spiritual is seen as superior it can lead to harmful attitudes that hinder a proper understanding of body, mind and spirit. At a superficial level such a misunderstanding encourages individuals to be 'so heavenly minded they are no earthly use' but, more significantly, this dualist approach can lead to spirituality becoming isolated from the rest of life. People who see the spiritual as superior may display negative attitudes towards what they consider physical – for example, women have sometimes been labelled as inferior because of their link with physical aspects of life such as childbirth. Paradoxically, while women may find their opportunities in religion restricted, they are often considered more spiritual than men. At the other extreme, those who value tangible physical and mental aspects of life above all else are given licence to ignore spirituality.

The exploratory group were particularly engaged by the sense that spirituality exists independently of any role (child, parent, professional) that a person adopts. We reflected together on the links and differences between the roles we adopted and our inner selves, and later developed this as a reflective activity that could be used in educational groups (as outlined in Box 5.4). In our discussions, we explored the idea of spirituality as the element that continues throughout our life, although it may be influenced by life events. One group member described it in this way:

> Through all the things you gain and lose throughout this journey, this period, there is a 'thing' that is with you and that is the essence of you and although that might change, you can't really lose that, it stays with you. So although

you lose lots of things and gain lots of things, that's a continuum in fact. There's a part of that child still within your spirituality.

Box 5.4 Imagine an onion

An onion has many layers, one within the other. Each layer is different yet is essentially part of the same onion. The layers are all connected to the root but not all can be seen from the outside. Imagine there are layers within you and consider the following comments and questions:

- Think about the roles or characteristics that are most visible on the surface, the most public parts of who you are, such as health carer, worker, parent. This is the layer of yourself that even strangers see.

- Under this public surface are attributes that fewer people see, starting with things that you are happy for friends and colleagues to know about, roles or abilities that people who know you in quite a public way will know. Think how other people might describe you (e.g. calm, cheerful, well organised) as well as what you do.

- What are the roles or attributes that lie under that surface, things that only a few people who are quite close to you will know about? These might be things about your upbringing or background as well as your present life, perhaps feelings or experiences you are anxious about or situations that leave you feeling vulnerable.

- Finally, how would you describe the internal heart of who you are, the person who exists within any external roles or abilities, perhaps that only you know about? This may include things that you even hesitate to admit to yourself.

All these layers are essentially you. Developing a greater awareness of the whole of you is part of spiritual awareness. There is no reason to share the most intimate knowledge of yourself with others but it is important to recognise what makes you who you are as this will affect you in many different ways.

Remembering and reflecting on people's life stories, as we found ourselves doing with clients and carers, helped identify what gave their lives meaning and purpose, connecting them with other people and with their worlds. The stories we heard, as well as those we told, provided a language and framework that helped interpret and shape those life events. Considering spirituality in this way suggests a connection with the past as well as a sense of life continuing into the future. We learned something of what made people who they were, the experiences and context that had made them uniquely themselves. This reflective process was important in our view of spirituality, helping identify and integrate what was of lasting value in an essentially personal exploration as if the essence of that person slowly emerged from its shelter. Such a view of spirituality could also provide a link to more communal or shared ideas that are embedded in someone's cultural and, sometimes, religious background.

Integrated yet transcendent

The idea of spirituality as a connecting or integrating force was also important to the group; we had already expressed our concern to ensure that spirituality was related to everyday experience as well as larger issues. We wanted to be able to discuss spirituality in terms of everyday tasks or relationships as well as reflect on the deep meaning of life. One group member noted how spirituality could be connected to something as mundane as ironing:

> People were very much making a big sort of distinction between the two and very much equating spirituality to the real deeper, big things…they were talking about women who wanted to talk about being about to do the ironing and [be] with the children. That it was very important to be the mummy and I felt that there was an element of spirituality within that … It's not being able to do the ironing, it's [who] they are, their role and their understanding of their role and purpose.

Our discussions emphasised the way in which spirituality was integral to the whole self, related to big questions about what it is to be human but also to roles and relationships in everyday life, indeed to every aspect of who we are. This emphasis complements the frequent suggestion that spirituality transcends everyday life, reaching out beyond the self to others, to a divine power or to absolute values such as love. Taken in isolation this can create the unhelpful impression that spirituality is separate from everyday life, again suggesting that spirituality is for only a particular type of person.

A more helpful emphasis that came up in the group was that spirituality integrated different dimensions of life, as illustrated in Figure 5.1: the human spirit draws together the horizontal in the sense of our connections and relationships with other people and with the world around us; and the vertical, in the sense of reaching out to transcendent meanings and, for some people, a divine being. We also discussed the idea of a third dimension, which involved reaching inward towards personal exploration, uniqueness and integration, another element referred to in writing about spirituality. A number of writers (for example, Giske 1995; Cobb and Robshaw 1998) refer to this multidimensional view of spirituality and we certainly found it a useful framework within which to explore ideas. An earlier discussion about the metaphor of weaving resurfaced as we considered how all these dimensions are interlinked to form one whole. One group discussed experiences with patients – for example, reflecting on the importance of family or friends in lifting someone's spirits or giving a sense of meaning and purpose. We talked at length about how one client had planned his own very special funeral in great detail with his family, using it to draw together some of the things that were important in his life. Planning it with him and later making sure it happened just as he wished made a connection between him and his family and friends that continued after his death in the immediate period of grief. The funeral was very practically linked to his life on Earth, his work and the people and places he had been connected to, but it also reached out to transcendent values, what lay beyond the bare facts of his life, what made these things important to him and how they gave meaning to his life and death.

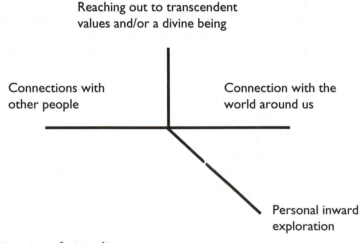

Figure 5.1 Dimensions of spirituality

Attempting to hold these different strands together as we considered spirituality in specific people or situations helped us understand that spirituality is not simply an isolated or internalised aspect of self but is, rather, earthed in everyday life. It also showed us how some aspects of spirituality can be more developed than others and helped us understand that spirituality exists whether or not it is recognised. Exploring and nurturing spirituality is a life-long process that simply occurs within the context of everyday life, provided there is some space and encouragement for that to happen. An interesting, even surprising, reflection of this is the inclusion of spirituality in discussions about the meaning and value of work. An investigation of the links between spirituality and work carried out by the Leeds Institute (Wilmer 1997) suggested that work was an important element in people's sense of meaning and purpose, and made a significant contribution to their life and spirituality. This should remind us to include the place of work when making a holistic assessment for individual patients or carers. In terms of health care practice this also suggests that spirituality needs to be considered as part of workforce development as well as patient care.

Nurturing spirituality

We came to realise that people should grow in spirit throughout their life span, just as we expect them to grow in body and mind. We would have been concerned if a person did not develop in these outward and visible ways, yet we rarely thought about someone's spiritual growth. We saw in our own lives, as well as in those of our clients, that the spiritual was often neglected and spiritual growth could be hindered by environmental or cultural factors. As we talked about spirituality, some people spoke of a sense of spiritual awakening that they could relate to particular incidents or experiences, at work or in other settings. Sometimes this was related to a spiritual experience rather like those described in Box 5.3 (p.88), others described the first experience of seeing someone die as profoundly influential. We were aware, though, that it was rare to talk to other people about such experiences. Opportunities to reflect on our own spiritual development with any sense of discernment seemed hard to find, not only because our lives are busy (when were they not?) but because this no longer seems a priority. This may be related to the lack of a familiar shared framework within which to nurture and explore spirituality. Whatever the difficulties of an imposed religious framework it did provide a starting point; church attendance at least offered space to sit and think in earlier busy lives. A new framework based round a much wider understanding of spirituality is described by the Kendal Project (Heelas and Woodhead 2005) but this is not yet widespread or robust enough to offer a universally agreed foundation for spirituality. In the groups I worked with, a shared framework emerged only slowly as we met to discuss and think about spirituality together.

Searching – for meaning, hope, connection or understanding – is an essential element of spiritual growth, supporting again the suggestion that 'the perpetual search for meaning in life' is the basis of spiritual existence (Cornette 1997, p.7). Spirituality seems to develop in encounters with life events, both positive and negative, rather than being something that is isolated from life experience. Writer Jennifer Lash describes her instinct to travel, both outwardly and inwardly, following her own experience of cancer:

> [Cancer] may be sharp and full of pain, but it may also be a guide, a useful companion on a dark night. There is a hidden current within every individual. It seeks and stirs, hides and yearns. Sometimes it is bewildered, a mixture of anger, pain and certainty. It may recede, but it never escapes. In moments of crisis, it is often full of voice. Make a Pilgrimage. Go to ancient places. Go wherever there are contemporary seekers. Go in whatever way it works out. Just go! (1998, p.xi)

Again this implies movement and the need to explore; spirituality, we were coming to realise, flourishes when there is this freedom to explore.

There are, of course, many ways of nurturing our own spirituality with different opportunities being important or available to people throughout their lives. A greater awareness of spirituality may help people access opportunities that are all around them, including the most ordinary activities. Taking time to be, to think or pray or just to be aware of the wonder of the world, all play their part in recognising and valuing spirituality in ourselves and others. It is hard to be aware of the inner world of the spirit in a busy, noisy environment where there seems little time to stop and reflect on anything. Realising the importance of spirituality can help individuals and teams recognise the benefit of protecting some quiet space for themselves and other people. Recognising that opportunities to be aware of spirituality are all around us became important in our discussions about spirituality; again we sensed that spirituality had to be recognised as an essential part of everyday experience rather than limited to rare events such as a meditation course or a trip abroad. There is a tacit recognition of the benefits of such personal development for health care staff, but people I worked with admitted that they rarely made time for it in their own work or leisure. Talking about spirituality together helped us understand what we might be missing as well as showing us more clearly how personal development might affect our work.

Whatever the needs of health care, if spirituality is innate it cannot in itself be taught. However, as with characteristics such as intelligence, sporting or musical ability, education offers an opportunity to develop and nurture that innate potential and the skills we need to nurture it in others. For example, listening to patients as they talk about spirituality is important and we can learn to listen better, to recognise and respond to tentative cues about spirituality. Many of the skills that health care professionals already have, such as communication skills and the ability to empathise, are of value once people recognise spirituality as an area in which these can be used. Similarly, if we acknowledge and are comfortable with our own innate spirituality, our own concerns or anxieties are less likely to stop us from hearing what people are saying about spirituality. Greater self-awareness about spirituality can help overcome a lack of confidence, enabling individuals to then use the skills and knowledge they already have more effectively.

The provision of an open and reflective environment creates opportunities where health care professionals can explore spirituality with other people in a way that is profoundly inclusive and enriching. That process creates a foundation on which to build, relating ideas about spirituality to the issues arising in people's personal lives and professional practice, and encouraging thoughtful consideration by individuals and the group. Although, in our group, we were gaining new knowledge and skills, even more important was the conscious reflection on our own spiritual life and health that underpinned any new understanding.

> You can learn particular skills, which will be effective to a limited degree, but it's very much the self work and from that realising how valuable this might be to you.

We were discovering that facing death or serious illness, as client, carer or health care worker, focuses attention on spirituality. When spirituality is understood in the broad way we have been describing, that link with health becomes even more apparent. Ill health can challenge individuals' sense of meaning and purpose, lead them to question values and beliefs, threaten or enhance relationships. Yet spiritual health is not contiguous with physical or mental health, although they are intimately connected. Illness, even life-threatening illness, is not necessarily associated with spiritual dis-ease. Group members reflected on how some clients whose physical health was deteriorating exhibited a sense of spiritual well-being, reminding us that spiritual growth may occur independently of physical health. Attending to their spirituality, through meditation, prayer or creative activities, is an important coping mechanism for some individuals but spirituality itself is much more than that. Again, Benson suggests that the best and most effective route to health and well-being relies on a balanced combination of medication, surgery or other procedures, and self-care (Benson with Stark 1996, p.23). A well-developed spirituality is a part of self-care, providing a necessary balance to physical and mental development, not separate from these other aspects of life but as much a part of well-being as they are. Indeed, it is the interaction between body, mind and spirit that really establishes health and well-being, with the human spirit exerting an influence on physical and mental health, and vice versa. A wide range of opportunities to explore and nurture spirituality, for those who wished to do so, became a key element in our understanding of spiritual care. We began to see spiritual care as providing a place where it was safe to reflect openly on spirituality within a holistic approach. This will be discussed further in the next chapter.

Talking about it

The human spirit, as we have described it, is that vital human spark, inseparable from the living physical body, that transcends physical need to speak of meaning, values and beliefs. Health care staff do not necessarily have the language or the confidence to reflect on the meaning of life at the same time as describing the efficacy of a particular treatment, however intimately these issues may be connected. This is not just a matter of skilful communication but is also about personal awareness and understanding of the issues involved. A number of key themes can be identified within much writing or discussion about spirituality in health care. These clusters of ideas about spirituality provide helpful openings from which to start exploring with clients or carers. Renetzky (1979) draws these ideas together when he describes spirituality as the fourth dimension: 'The power within a person's life that gives meaning, purpose and fulfilment; the will to live; the belief or faith that person has in self, in others and in a power beyond self' (p.215).

Couched in language less 'slippery' (Jenkins 1997) than spirituality itself, ideas about meaning and purpose, connection, hope and religion can provide opportunities for health care teams to approach an issue that is frequently difficult to discuss.

Meaning, purpose and hope

Walter (1997, p.25) reviews three different approaches to spiritual care in palliative medicine, finally identifying the search for meaning as advantageous in most settings. As referred to earlier, Cicely Saunders, the pioneer of the modern hospice movement, has been influential in promoting this approach to spirituality, which draws on Viktor Frankl's idea of logotherapy or a therapy of meaning (Frankl 1964). Frankl recognised the importance of having a sense of meaning during his experience in the concentration camps of the Second World War and used these ideas subsequently in his work as a psychiatrist. Although the meaning of life suggests an overarching or ultimate purpose rather remote from everyday concerns, Frankl is clear that there are many sources of meaning, including love, beauty, creativity, relationships, religious beliefs and even pleasure. Gardener and writer Monty Don has suggested that everyday activities have in fact become doubly precious in the aftermath of the 11 September 2001 terrorist attacks in New York:

> I have no embarrassment about elevating the goals and rewards of gardening to the spiritual. It seems self evident in the sheer power of the life force that fills every cell of the smallest backyard to the great estates. The trick is to pay attention to it, to notice things, to be fully alive yourself. (2001, p.74)

The groups of health care staff I worked with were certainly aware of more everyday aspects of meaning found, for example, in the relationships or tasks that help people cope with life. We have already talked about how household tasks, such as ironing, can be a reflection of people's role and contribute to their sense of who they are. In my own work as a dietitian I had seen how concerns about eating or weight change are related to wider concerns such as the loss of purpose experienced by someone who can no longer cook for the family or who no longer enjoys food. Discussions about the ultimate meaning and purpose of human existence merged into these more everyday discussions; this fluidity linked well with the idea that spirituality should relate to everyday concerns as well as deeper issues.

The sense of meaning can also be linked with having hope, not only the obvious hope of a cure for those who are ill but also in a much wider sense. Hope may be embedded in human relationships and the sense of life continuing through others. Many clients described their hopes that their life would be made meaningful by their influence on other people or on situations. Perhaps this is more easily seen where clients have children or grandchildren who carry forward their physical genes as well as their ideas and memory. However, many people talked of their hope that their influence would continue through other people in the wider community of work and society. We noticed how we too experienced this sense of someone's life continuing through the effect clients had on our own ideas. We remembered them and passed those memories on to others, particularly where individuals had influenced our own practice. As we told their stories, in teaching sessions or contact with other clients, there was a sense that their lives were continuing and had not been without meaning. This sense of purpose and hope in the future can have a very positive impact on health and well-being. A strong sense of meaning and hope supports people as they cope with difficult experiences and contributes to overall well-being or even recovery. Frankl described how individuals in the concentration camps who kept hope alive and retained a sense of purpose seemed to survive better (1964, p.35).

Our own experiences suggested that people's ability to cope with treatment and illness was, at least in part, influenced by such factors. A powerful pull towards well-being was exerted by the desire, for example, to see a new grandchild or a family wedding. It was also true that clients who seemed to lose all hope appeared to struggle more and perhaps fail to cope with treatment. Hope is a complex issue in health care; health care professionals are, rightly, concerned not to give false hope yet it seems important to help clients to retain a sense of hope. Certainly, talking about people's sense of hope is another place where questions about spirituality are raised and it is important that health care professionals are open to that opportunity.

Perhaps spiritual growth is, in part, about developing a sense of meaning that relates to the whole of life, difficulty and pain as well as joy and ease. This suggests that spirituality will develop in encounters with life events rather than separated from them. If spirituality is a movement towards wholeness, it adds weight to the importance of 'a living connection between the surface and the unfathomable and meaning rich depths of who we are' (Kearney 1996, p.59). Understanding spirituality as a positive aspect of health – well-being, not just struggle – reinforces the sense that this is a common human task rather than something that is relevant only to a small number of seriously ill clients.

Some research does support the idea that spirituality can have a positive influence on health and well-being although much more work is needed. The evidence base for the NICE guidelines on supportive and palliative care for adults with cancer (King's College London 2004) gives some examples with the cautionary recognition that findings remain preliminary. Other specific examples from different areas of health care include: a connection between spiritual awareness and well-being in a survey of terminally ill, hospitalised adults (Reed 1987); a link between social support, active problem solving, and life satisfaction and spirituality in people with HIV/AIDS, particularly in non-white women (Somali and Heckman 2000); the emergence of spirituality (identified as prayer, meditation, religious practices or belief in God) as a powerful coping force in breast cancer survivors (Fredette 1995); the importance of religious beliefs and the supportive religious communities for some people with mental health problems (Health Education Authority 1999; Swinton 2001). Other examples of a positive link between spirituality and well-being are summarised in Post, Puchalski and Larson (2000). Such a potentially positive force deserves to be recognised by health care professionals in parallel with the knowledge that serious illness may precipitate a spiritual crisis, particularly when the individual's sense of purpose and worth are affected. For example, a survey reporting low levels of spiritual distress among people with lung cancer, noted that greater distress was experienced by young people and by those who felt less physically well (Highfield 1992, p.7). Spiritual distress may be more likely where people appear to have lost touch with their sense of meaning, but predicting whose sense of meaning will be most challenged is not easy. Awareness of spirituality in every person and setting is therefore even more important.

The groups I was involved with all highlighted the importance of trying to make sense of life experiences as important in its own right even if no over-arching meaning was found. This links again with the sense of spirituality as 'the perpetual search for meaning in life' (Cornette 1997, p.7) and a description by Simsen, a nurse researching spirituality, that the search for meaning is like 'the border in a jigsaw puzzle' (1986, p.42), giving shape and boundaries to our lives. Our own experience of exploring spirituality together highlighted the fact that within our professional roles we were still human beings with our own needs for understanding, meaning and purpose. We came to see that opportunities for reflection, individually and with others, were an important part of this lifelong process, part of our own spiritual growth as well as that of our clients, a place where we and they could try to make sense of life experiences. Struggling to describe the process of spiritual care, one participant put it this way:

> There are times when you find a lost soul, and I don't mean that in a religious sense or anything, but someone who hasn't come to terms…with life or death… They haven't had the time or the energy to think about the meaning

of life for them and suddenly they're…faced with a life-threatening disease, they're thrown into the crisis of what life is all about.

Far from trying to create meaning for such clients, the role of health care staff is to provide support while people explore the significance of past and current experiences to develop their own sense of meaning. In the end the meaning someone draws from a particular experience is unique but the process of seeking meaning is something human beings share. Understanding and valuing this process in ourselves helps health care professionals recognise and value it for their clients as well as each other.

Connection

The idea of spirituality as a sense of connection links with some of the underlying concepts discussed earlier, such as integration. Certainly, the idea of connection was a frequent discussion point in the groups I worked with, sometimes appearing to act as a summary for ideas about the nature of spirituality. We recognised the importance of a sense of connection with other people in our own personal development; relationships with people (clients or others) affected us in so many ways, drawing us out of our self-absorption and contributing to our sense of meaning. Relationships with family or friends reminded us we were not alone in the universe but part of a greater whole. Many of those involved in exploring spirituality could describe relationships with clients that had had a particular influence on their thinking and development. This greater sense of connection developed with some clients, those we could relate to but also those with whom we felt we had shared a period of struggle or difficulty. Of course, our care extended beyond the few individuals where there was a specific sense of connection to the wider community of our clients, but these more focused experiences of connection were often highly significant. It would be impossible to experience a close connection with every client; we were also conscious that such experiences had to be handled with care in order to ensure a fair and equitable service.

Connection is about more than human relationships, however – there is also the sense of an internal connection, as described earlier, and for some people a link with a divine presence or with the Earth, as in the descriptions of spiritual experience outlined earlier. These were all factors that people recognised as elements of spirituality, which had shaped and nurtured our own individual spirituality. With hindsight, I felt the groups I was working with used the term 'connection' in two quite different ways and did not always distinguish between them. Connection in spiritual care was seen as both a particular feeling of closeness with a few specific clients and a more general concept within our understanding of spirituality. It was helpful to recognise both aspects of this idea of connection and to be aware how it might affect us.

Religion

Although religion has links with spirituality the two are not synonymous, as is still often assumed. Religion, at best, should always be spiritual but spirituality may have little or no religious connection. Rather, spirituality can be understood as the broader concept, a potential within all human beings that is concerned, as we have already discussed, with connection, meaning, hope and other metaphysical concerns. Religion is better viewed as a particular system of faith and worship (Little *et al.* 1973); for some people this provides an important way of expressing their spirituality, but it is certainly not the only way and not for everyone.

While there is now a greater recognition that religion and spirituality are not synonymous, the link between spirituality and religion in health care is still strong. Reviewing the nursing literature in 1978, Kreidler found that in most cases the word 'spirituality' was equated with religion (quoted in Labun 1988, p.314) and more recent writers note that spirituality is still commonly linked with religion (for example, Highfield and Cason 1983, p.189; Burnard 1990, p.38; Ross, 1994, p.442).

Individuals involved in the exploring spirituality groups were uncomfortable with a purely religious understanding of spirituality, feeling this was inappropriate for an open care centre where the staff themselves did not share a common faith. In Walter's (1997) review of three different approaches to spiritual care, he suggests that recognising spirituality as a broad concept linked to meaning is particularly helpful for centres such as ours that do not have a particular religious framework or community. Ideas about meaning and purpose, connection and hope were more open and acceptable entry points to begin discussing spirituality. However, it is noteworthy that all the groups I worked with spent a significant amount of time discussing religion, including differing experiences of religion and belief.

Religion, then, should not be ignored but rather understood as a way of expressing spirituality that remains important for many people. Religious needs in health care should not be neglected or stereotyped as interest in spirituality grows. Within any faith community there will be a range of different interpretations about how that faith should be lived out. Chaplains from different faith communities play a vital role in supporting people in their religious needs but the wider health care team also needs to help ensure these are not neglected. Some religious practices – for example, dress or behaviour – provide measurable opportunities to record how this aspect of spirituality affects the lives of individuals but this should be recognised as the tip of an iceberg. Religious practice, rather than spirituality, may be monitored in health surveys simply because it is easier to measure. We have already discussed how religion is important to people in hospital, recognising that religious requirements for prayer, worship, particular food or privacy should be recognised and provided for (Simsen 1986, p.42; Ross 1997b, p.713). Religious practice retains greater cultural significance for older people and those with a non-European background (Royal College of Nursing Resource Guide 1998, p.8). For some people, previously dormant religious beliefs become more important in illness, highlighting the wider requirements for privacy, quiet and respect in health care settings of all types. Spiritual and religious beliefs may still be overlooked by health services, including mental health and children's services, despite their importance to some service users. A report in 1999, based on research by the National Schizophrenia Fellowship, proposed a positive role for faith communities in promoting mental health, particularly through social support and links with a wider community (Health Education Authority 1999; Swinton 2001).

Members of specific faith communities are generally understood to have a range of overlapping beliefs and practices that centre around a common framework that affects individuals and communities. Berger (1969, p.38) used the term 'sacred canopy' to suggest how religion creates a community of shared values or a particular way of viewing the world. This canopy protects and legitimises shared meanings held by religious communities in a wider frame of reference. Like spirituality, religion is concerned with recurring human themes such as creation, life and death, and hope. Religious institutions tend to formalise belief and practice in a way that may restrict spiritual growth but, conversely, religious structures can foster such growth by providing a communal discipline and structure rather than relying purely on individual preferences or experience. Such a supportive but diverse community can challenge beliefs that are potentially damaging for individuals or groups (such as racism, extreme asceticism) although, sadly, extreme religious groups may also encourage or impose harmful beliefs – for example, mass suicides or aggression towards others. Providing a challenging but supportive community in which to explore ideas and beliefs is not so very different from what our exploratory groups were doing!

Conclusion

A clearer understanding of spirituality helps all health care staff to respond appropriately to anyone (religious or not) who wishes to explore spiritual issues. Meeting religious needs (for example, for sacraments or particular food) is an important organisational issue and there is a clear role for chaplaincy services (and other staff) in recognising and responding effectively to these religious needs. However, if spirituality is defined purely in terms of religion, non-religious clients will be excluded while the broader spiritual needs of all clients may remain unrecognised. Much of the current public interest in spirituality lies outside any of the major faith communities, linked, for example, to new-age groups, alternative communities, the women's movement and environmental organisations, as outlined by the Kendal Project (Heelas and Woodhead 2005). For example, a review of spirituality and the secular quest (Van Ness 1996) showed many non-religious ways in which spirituality can be expressed, including sport, the Arts, and social issues such as feminism, justice, health and ecology. Spirituality provides a convenient, non-religious way of reminding people that there is still more to life than the physical and material, and this transcendent element of human nature, whatever we call it, can be expressed in many ways including, for example, poetry, art and music. This understanding in turn helps create a view of spiritual care and how it can be provided in practice.

Ultimately the groups with which I worked wanted a way of exploring spirituality that would make a difference to their practice both as individuals and in the teams where we worked. The time we spent exploring the nature of spirituality together was an essential preparation for incorporating our ideas about spirituality into our practice. This is not an area where outline theoretical ideas can simply be adopted wholesale but rather those ideas, and our own response to them, have to be teased out and interpreted according to our experience. They then become a part of who we are and how we work. Perhaps the difficulty of that process is the real reason why spirituality remains so neglected in health care. Our experience suggests that once the process has started it offers an opening for health care teams to consider what can be offered as the spiritual element of the holistic approach.

6

Spiritual Care

Earlier chapters have already made clear that the increasing interest in spirituality, both generally and within health care, does not necessarily affect actual health care practice. Yet it seems clear that contact with illness, particularly life-threatening illness, is a time when people become more aware of spiritual concerns. Illness may stop people doing the very things that give them a sense of meaning and purpose, destroy their hopes for the future or damage their connections with family and friends; all these, and more, affect their understanding of who they are and what they are about. Clients and carers alike may want to explore these changes within the context of health care; this exploration may affect what health care is required or acceptable. Yet the evidence we have suggests such spiritual needs are not always recognised or responded to, at least in part because of misunderstanding about the nature and provision of spiritual care. Opportunities for health care teams to explore spirituality together are essential in establishing a setting in which people who are ill can receive spiritual care, and staff can provide it, safely and effectively. Spiritual care, then, is essentially about providing a safe and hospitable place where people can choose to explore spirituality in the way that suits them best. As one writer puts it:

> Optimal spiritual health may be considered as the ability to develop our spiritual nature to its fullest potential. This would include our ability to discover and articulate our own basic purpose in life, learn how to experience love, joy, peace and fulfilment and how to help ourselves and others achieve their fullest potential. (Chapman 1986, p.41)

Quite a tall order for anyone!

The experience of people I worked with supports research suggesting that spiritual care is more likely to be provided by people who have a personal understanding of spirituality. Hence it is important that opportunities to explore spirituality within the team create links with personal and professional experience as well as theoretical ideas. Talking about spirituality to other team members builds confidence and enables the whole team to develop an integrated approach based on a shared understanding of spirituality. The process of learning to understand spirituality together equips individuals to provide spiritual care on behalf of the whole team. Working within a team that shares an understanding of spirituality also ensures there is support for individual team members in this area. Only then can health care teams become the sort of safe and hospitable places where spiritual care is provided in ways that suit the needs of differing clients.

Establishing a context for spiritual care

Where spiritual concerns are recognised in health care, two main factors are thought to prevent staff, usually nursing staff, from responding: first, the perception that spiritual care is the realm of the hospital chaplain; and second, a sense of being unable to respond for a variety of personal and professional reasons, including a lack of appropriate education (see, for example, Oldnall 1996, p.142; Ross 1997a, pp.40–1). Nursing staff of all grades are in a prime position to recognise and respond to spiritual concerns but there is no reason to suppose other professional groups within the health care team should not also be involved. Allied health professionals, such as occupational therapists, physiotherapists, speech and language therapists and dietitians, will also be in a position to listen and respond when particular patients express concerns that touch on such spiritual issues. Some areas may also wish to involve the wider team in their response, including volunteers or other therapists. Support staff, as we have already discussed, make a significant contribution to spiritual care in some ward areas and, again, may be the ones who hear patient concerns. We have already discussed, in Chapter 3, how members of the health care team may be involved in spiritual care and support in different ways while still working within a common framework, and effective education about spirituality is essential in order to equip them for that task.

As the groups I worked with explored spirituality and spiritual care, they recognised how talking about spirituality with each other made it easier to talk to people outside our group, including clients and carers. We first became aware of, and then learnt to overcome, barriers that had previously prevented us exploring the whole topic of spirituality. We became more sensitive to this issue and more confident, more able to listen and respond when clients raised spiritual concerns. We were less anxious when spiritual concerns seemed to be looming; we were more comfortable knowing that our role was not to resolve such concerns. That left us free to stay with people as they explored, to encourage and accept this process rather than block or ignore it. In this way a broad range of health care professionals within our multi-professional team was equipped to respond appropriately when clients raised spiritual issues. A shared foundation also makes it easier, even safer, to be proactive; when spirituality was openly recognised as part of the health care team's work there were natural opportunities for clients to explore this aspect of themselves if they wished to do so.

Educational opportunities that enable health care teams to explore spirituality in this personal and reflective way are clearly an important aspect of spiritual care as they underpin and support more practical activities. Philosophical discussions about the nature of spirituality and spiritual care may appear to be quite abstract elements of the spiritual journey but these are inseparably bound to the most practical and earthy elements of health care provision. Embedding health care within the holistic approach ensures that even discussions about the most intimate physical care occur within a framework of respect and attention to the whole person that is essentially spiritual. For example, a nurse in one educational group reflected how her conversation with a client moved seamlessly from questions about loss and grief to a very practical discussion about bowel care. Her new-found awareness of spirituality increased her confidence to listen and respond appropriately throughout, recognising all aspects of this conversation as relevant to spirituality and untangling them only where necessary. Another member of the original discussion group spoke of how talk about coping strategies had led naturally into talk about spirituality, moving on again to discuss connections with family and friends. Similar experiences in our own discussions had alerted us to the way that spirituality wove in and out of wide-ranging aspects of health and well-being.

Given the way in which spirituality has been sidelined in modern culture, the chance to have a non-confrontational, exploratory discussion about spirituality is now fairly rare, so it is not surprising that clients and health care professionals alike find it difficult to articulate and explore this area. Health care professionals need excellent communication skills to support clients through this process but, even more importantly, they also need to be comfortable with their own personal understanding and experiences of spirituality.

There is a real danger of making spiritual care something else we *do to* clients rather than something that is essentially about being human, about who we all are more than what we do. Spiritual care must never become simply another box to tick.

The whole process of exploring such an integral aspect of holistic care is also an opportunity to build team understanding and support, touching as it does on so many different aspects of health care. The development of consensus and an overarching understanding about something as personal and extensive as spirituality is not simple. It requires team members to hear and value personal and professional experience (their own and other people's) in a way that fosters a deep understanding and respect for each other. It also requires them to reflect in quite a challenging way on aspects of themselves and their work, aspects they currently accept without thinking. This shared understanding, elements of which are discussed in the previous chapter, sets the scene for the provision of spiritual care. Without sharing this underpinning framework, it is surely a mistake even to try to impose the provision of spiritual care on individual members of the multi-professional health care team. Individuals involved in providing spiritual care need to be able to absorb and integrate ideas about spirituality for themselves to make such provision possible. While this may all seem rather slow, in practice once the process has started, learning about and providing spiritual care flow naturally together. Understanding continues to grow as people's reflections on their experience of spiritual care begin to be discussed more openly within the team. This is, after all, an area where lifelong learning certainly applies and no one has all the answers.

The nature of spiritual care

Religious activities, meditation, outdoor pursuits, expressive and creative arts, all provide potential avenues through which individuals may express or explore their spirituality. The groups with which I worked already had access to a number of such activities within the working environment, including gardening, art, meditation, music and creative writing, as well as a wide range of complementary therapies; some of these were open to staff as well as clients and carers. Superficially, expanding the range of these opportunities appeared to be the best way of providing spiritual care within the workplace. Yet, as we discussed this further, it became clear that all these activities, although an extremely valuable resource, were not in themselves the essence of spiritual care. There is something to be learned by considering what spiritual care is not. For example, this speaker refers to a discussion the group had about a particular paper on spiritual care:

> The thing is…they were sort of talking about creativity being a spiritual thing. They were talking about diversional activities. I think there's much more [to it] than that and I just got a bit irritated. I felt what they were doing was to kind of highlight the idea of what is spiritual and then look round to see 'Ah yes, well what have we got? Oh yes, that's quite spiritual.'

In the same way, spirituality is not only concerned with basic requirements for privacy and dignity, including quiet space, respect for personal beliefs and values, important as these are for all aspects of holistic health care. Opportunities to explore and clarify the team's understanding of spirituality help distinguish the actual essence of spirituality from other related aspects of health care.

Spiritual care is often assumed, consciously or unconsciously, to be the same as religious care, something we have already disputed. This distinction between religion and spirituality is not intended to reduce the value of religion; sociological evidence suggests that religion remains important to significant numbers of people in Britain, particularly older people and those with a non-European background (Davie and Cobb 1998, p.89). Despite the decline in church attendance, nominal religious allegiance continues to exert a widespread and sometimes subtle influence on people's lives. Religious needs – for example, for particular food or rites – should not be ignored by health services, and there is a clear and important role for multi-faith chaplaincy services in recognising and responding to these religious needs. For some clients religious and spiritual beliefs will always be intertwined; for others previously dormant religious beliefs become more important in illness. All health care staff need to honour these religious needs and understand how to respond when they recognise them in individual clients. Yet where those same health care staff continue to assume that all spiritual care has a religious basis then non-religious clients will be excluded and the broader spiritual needs of all clients will be forgotten.

Psychological support is also sometimes confused with spiritual care, perhaps not surprisingly when spiritual, psychological and physical well-being are very much intertwined in the holistic approach. Supportive activities, including counselling or psychological support, are all extremely important elements of mental health care; although not in themselves spiritual, there is bound to be overlap with spiritual care, and physical care, when looking at a holistic approach. Spiritual and/or religious beliefs may be overlooked by mental health services, yet a psychological crisis may prompt an exploration of spirituality in a similar way to a physical crisis. There is increasing aware-ness of the need to recognise religious and spiritual care within mental health services. Ignoring spiritual or religious needs can mean that vital opportuni-ties to work with clients are lost; for example, some faith communities make a very positive contribution to mental health care services, particularly around integration with the wider community (Health Education Authority 1999).

So, if spiritual care is not about a particular activity, how can it best be described? The metaphor of the search or journey that has provided a recur-ring theme in our discussions about spirituality so far can also provide a model for health care, including spiritual care. Highfield (1997, p.237) describes a well-mapped cancer journey through diagnosis, treatment, remission, mainte-nance, recurrence and survival or death. The outward journey through disease, often marked by rough and difficult terrain, stimulates in some people a parallel inner journey. It seems superfluous to state the importance of the outer journey that provides the stimulus for this other exploration, but there is a danger in concentrating on it too much. This tunnel vision means that health care staff fail to recognise that the outer journey does not encompass the whole of life nor is it necessarily, in the end, the most important part of the route. Health care workers who concentrate their efforts on recognisable physical signs and symptoms may miss the important underlying journey with which their clients are also engaged. It is this journey, more than the outer one, that will enable people to begin to make sense of their life, perhaps leading to changes in activity or outlook as they re-evaluate what is important to them. That process will inevitably affect health care, not only clients' decisions about treatment and response to it but also their sense of well-being.

Ultimately each individual makes his or her own spiritual journey and the provision of spiritual care can be understood as walking with someone on that journey. When they provide spiritual care, health care staff may find them-selves joining that journey as a companion, not a spiritual guide but someone who acknowledges and respects each individual's life journey and may pro-vide support and companionship on the way.

> Perhaps the journey is the thing we all have in common, that we are all, not just us but all people, potentially on a journey, whether they have elected to start travelling or not…and there's something about how we journey alongside other people.

This supports the idea that spiritual care is more about being than doing, about who we are rather than the tasks we carry out. Health care staff who acknowledge and encourage their own spiritual journey are likely to understand and respond to this better. Creative activities, including music, art and writing, provide helpful opportunities to express emotional and spiritual needs without words, as well as to discover new abilities and enjoyment, but they remain supportive activities rather than encompassing the whole of spiritual care. It may be that no activities or specific support are required, yet simply by recognising and honouring a client's spirituality health care staff have provided spiritual care of the most profound sort. Attending to the whole person, including the spiritual dimension, has the potential to facilitate a deeper and more complete healing than physical care in isolation:

> Spiritual care seeks to nurture the inner self and the framework of meanings and values through which it is expressed. It also aims to sustain people through the shadow side of their personality, the alien within, that emerges during periods of great stress and grief. (Amenta 1997, p.4)

Discussions with other colleagues supported this sense that a commitment to our own inner journey was an essential preparation for journeying with others. The shared exploration of spirituality considered here provides one approach to this preparation, not the only one by any means but a significant reminder for anyone working in health care that his or her own spiritual life should not be neglected. It is important to remember also that this process poses significant challenges for busy health care professionals, which will be discussed later.

Being not doing

Simply relieving pain and distress, as would be natural with a physical problem, is not necessarily the answer in spiritual care. Health care staff should not attempt to sort out clients' personal spiritual struggles but rather support them as they undertake this process for themselves. We need to find a different way of providing spiritual care, a way of being rather than doing, which acknowledges that spiritual care is more about who we are than what we do:

> If I were to…shout out to a nurse or a doctor, you know, 'Don't just stand there, do something' but in fact what's crying out in many people is, you know, 'Don't do something, just stand there,' you know…and there aren't any rule books for that…Well, the strategy is to be human.

High-quality, evidence-based, technical advice and treatment is vital for effective health care; complementary therapies and psychosocial support are also important elements of care but none of these encompasses the whole of health care. Elements of spiritual care should also be subject to rational consideration and review – for example, as seen in the evidence for the NICE guidelines (King's College London 2004), which include recent research about spiritual care in adults with cancer. However, the research review itself includes a warning against medicalising spiritual concerns: 'Spiritual care can become transformed into a rational discourse of measurement, diagnosis and audit' (King's College London 2004, p.175). Although less measurable, attitudes to people, including the respect with which they are treated and the time and attention they receive, are as important as technical treatment and support. An understanding of spirituality supports this need to recognise and respond to people as human beings, including the recognition that health care providers are human too. Clients and health care staff are involved in health care for different reasons; they have different needs and abilities that should not be forgotten. Spirituality is a reminder that, despite these differences, we are still all fellow human beings. A sense of shared and equal humanity underpins the provision of spiritual care, supporting empathy, understanding and acceptance.

The very essence of spirituality is about being human, with the spiritual lived out through an intricate web of physical, mental and social life so that this sense of the transcendent weaves through the whole of life. It should be no surprise, then, that simply being human, rather than any particular activity or task, is at the heart of spiritual care. Rather than being a role we play or a task we carry out, in spiritual care who we are makes an implicit contribution throughout all our health care provision. The compassion and empathy that is offered, the attitude that gives hope or believes in someone or that makes a human connection, are the result of this human-to-human relationship; elements of all health care, they may be more easily recognised in spiritual care. Being human sounds straightforward but in practice it is harder and more demanding than many more technical aspects of care. Some people seem to bring this positive human element into their work as naturally as breathing and would probably be bemused to be asked how this happens.

> I think…we all have an inherent quality within us which we can hone, we can fine-tune, we can learn skills to focus in on. Certain people will be able to work with other people or will connect with other people for whatever reason but I don't think you can learn to be real, I think you can unlearn all the things that stop you being real.

I wonder if the process of professional training contributes to the difficulty that some health care professionals find with this human connection. Perhaps the very process of learning to act in a professional role makes it harder to remember the essential humanity we share with each other and with our clients. The human dimension of spiritual care reminds us of that shared humanity and may seem to transcend professional boundaries. Any such crossing of these boundaries must be treated with caution simply because they are intended to protect both health care professionals and their clients. We learn, of necessity, to distance ourselves from too frequent and painful reminders of our own human-ness; we must also learn to protect the client from seeing our own pain or fears. Somehow within this necessary protective process we need to remember that we are human and acknowledge that being human can be painful and difficult, yet we must find a way to do that without harming our clients or ourselves. As one person described it:

> Spirituality isn't like anything else because it isn't a technique you can learn, it isn't a theory you can learn, it isn't a psychological approach, it isn't an analytical approach. It is in fact about sharing something of you, which, although at the best anybody that is helping anybody should be sharing something of themselves, but this is a much more vulnerable, open uncharted area, isn't it?

Learning, almost re-learning, what it is to be human in practice is an important element of becoming an established and experienced professional. Such a person provides excellent technical care as well as that essential human connection that somehow embodies spiritual care. Greater self-awareness is part of that process, helping avoid unacknowledged feelings and attitudes having a negative effect on patient care as well as increasing awareness of who we are, including our own spiritual life. The reflective, rather philosophical, discussions about spirituality and spiritual care described so far are intended to connect this implicit concern simply to bring ourselves into our health care practice with a helpful level of personal and professional understanding. Of course, talking about spirituality will not in itself achieve that sort of connection but it can be a positive part of the process. Talking to other members of the health care team about spirituality requires team members to make themselves vulnerable and to be open about their own difficulties as well as listening to others, and that is surely a good place to start. It should also provide a base for the necessary continuing support that will be needed by staff who engage in this process.

Spirituality, that most intangible aspect of health care, can be seen in many different ways when health care staff treat people as whole beings. Not all of these are about doing more activity, mostly they are about the way in which any activity is done. Taking time, listening, valuing and respecting people are all part of this approach to care and can be seen in the most practical of activities. Examples would be the carer who sees beyond the present frail and vulnerable client to the person who was once strong and confident, and remembers that he or she is the same person; the team member who listens and tries to understand how a particular treatment feels to a client then brings that understanding into his or her work; the staff member who treats someone with dignity and respect through the most intimate of procedures. Thinking more widely, organisations demonstrate this approach when they try to take account of the patient's perspective, attend to the effects of the environment on the whole person, or support staff development. In all these ways holistic care is wordlessly being provided and I suspect that remembering the spiritual, that essential intangible shared human-ness, underpins such provision. This approach can be difficult to sustain within the current emphasis on evidence-based practice despite the support for a holistic approach, yet excellent technical care will never be enough without it.

The inclusion of personal spirituality when preparing health care staff for involvement in spiritual care is a massive challenge. Talking to others about personal beliefs and values is always hazardous; such openness can be misinterpreted or treated with disdain by colleagues who are themselves struggling to express their own beliefs and values. Talking about spirituality reminds us, we have said, of our own vulnerability, and health care professionals familiar with a helping role often struggle to accept their own helplessness in the face of a client's struggle. The 'busyness' of doing something when we deal with more practical issues can divert attention from this underlying reluctance and there is always plenty to do. There is a recognised need for training in basic skills that enable the recognition of spiritual need and provision of spiritual or religious support (School of Health and Related Research 2004, p.39). For some individuals within the health care team this will be enough but it feels incomplete to consider spirituality without any recognition of personal spirituality and how that affects work in health care. The general perplexity about spirituality leaves people – health care professionals and their clients – ill equipped to reflect on such questions of identity, meaning and hope. Again as one of our group noted:

> We spend so little time even throwing ideas out, you know, 'That truth's not for me and that truth's not for me.' Yes, we can say 'I'm a moral person' and 'I love my neighbour and I get on with my life,' but we don't really spend a lot of time, as people, talking about [spirituality]. Not necessarily to seek anything or to come up with any answers but at least spend time exploring it.

I think so many people go through their life and never do and I think that's a shame.

An opportunity to do some of this reflection in a health care context, especially with others who are struggling with similar issues and experiences, can only help health care professionals support their clients more effectively in this area.

Spiritual support

There are many sources of spiritual support, including friends, family or religious groups, and the multi-professional groups I worked with were keen to acknowledge and utilise this range. However, our experience suggested that clients who raised concerns about spiritual issues often seemed to lack other sources of spiritual support. A general lack of clarity about the nature of spirituality, plus the difficulties already described of raising the topic, may mean that support is not available or is not seen as relevant to the issues involved. If someone has largely ignored spirituality previously, it is perhaps not surprising that they lack support structures in this area. We increasingly saw a role in ensuring that clients are offered opportunities to talk about spiritual issues within health care. Of course, clients may not wish to explore their spiritual concerns at all, or at least not within that setting, and must retain their right to reject spiritual support or to explore spirituality in the way they choose. Our concern was to make sure that spirituality was not neglected or ignored but openly part of our remit to provide holistic care. Where health care teams adopt a broad understanding of spirituality, spiritual care can be understood as creating a safe and hospitable space in which clients can attend to their spirit in the way that is important to them. Their choices about spiritual support may be very different from those of the health care professionals working with them, but that does not mean that spiritual care has not been provided. In such an environment, clients are able to reflect on the spiritual questions their experience raises, both positive and negative. Health care staff need to be equipped to support them in this process, including understanding when and how to refer them to other sources of spiritual or religious support if required.

The therapeutic relationship

Underlying this approach to spiritual care is the recognition that positive relationships between health care professionals and clients are a vital element of health care rather than an optional extra. Such therapeutic relationships are founded on Carl Rogers' core conditions of genuineness, acceptance and empathy (Mearns and Thorne 1999, pp.16, 22) and provide an appropriate context for spiritual care. This approach emphasises both the centrality of the client and the supportive role of the health care professional; it returns to the idea of the journey, with health care professionals travelling alongside their clients for a time. Rather than take clients to a particular goal, Jean Vanier, founder of the L'Arche communities, suggests that our task is more like learning their language (in Stoter 1995, p.27).

The core conditions of the therapeutic relationship provide an environment where spiritual concerns can safely be probed by clients as part of their own growth towards wholeness. Remembering spirituality helps health care professionals avoid slipping into an essentially technical approach to health, particularly with the current emphasis on effectiveness, standards and audit. Intrinsically human to human, spiritual care is based on a partnership that recognises the shared humanity of clients and health care professionals. Such a partnership affects all aspects of their care, ensuring that clients are no longer just patients but people. Providing spiritual care is not only about recognising and responding to spiritual questions but also about an essential respect for the human spirit and its potential. This very human dimension of health care is the essence of spiritual care and should infuse all elements of our activity.

The health care professionals I worked with recognised the common ground they shared with clients: we too struggled to find meaning in life; to explore unanswerable metaphysical questions; to connect with other people and to reach out to transcendent values. This is not to discount our professional skills, simply to recognise their limitations; we have no cure to offer for spiritual distress, we can only offer ourselves and, realistically, we are not always able to offer that. In this way, spiritual care requires a level of openness and vulnerability, a recognition of our own needs as well as those of our clients, that challenges professional expertise and brings a certain humility. We recognised instances where we had received more in terms of spirituality from clients than we had been able to give – the physically diseased offering their spiritual strength to support the physically well. This reversal may save health care professionals from the tyranny of a curative medical model where we must make everything better or we have failed; it also reminds us that the balance of power in professional relationships may become distorted if the client is no longer paramount.

The cost of spiritual care

The clear benefits of using a holistic approach in health care are discussed elsewhere, and the spiritual dimension is an integral part of this approach. Spiritual care has a cost like any other aspect of health care; that is not a reason to exclude this essential and beneficial element of health care but such costs must still be counted.

We could start with the seemingly simple cost of providing spiritual care: the use of facilities, including adequate space and time, as well as the need for specialist staff and appropriate training (School of Health and Related Research 2004, pp.38–42). Even more important, though, is the emotional cost of personal involvement in spiritual care, including recognising our own limitations. A clearer understanding of spirituality and spiritual care should enrich clients and health care professionals alike, ensuring both are recognised and treated as unique, whole human beings, but it also places demands on vulnerable health care professionals who must be protected from burn-out when the demands upon them become too great. Engaging in holistic care challenges our own values or beliefs, and that too may have a spiritual cost, perhaps ultimately enriching, but also potentially deeply disturbing.

Yet exploring spirituality is not without benefits to weigh against these costs. Encouraging individuals to attend to their own spirit is an important way of maintaining health and well-being among staff. Hall, a nurse working with people living with HIV, suggests that this process is part of 'learning to be ourselves – authentically and with confidence' (1997, p.90). Considering their own spirituality may lead staff to develop a more connected approach in their own lives, realising the benefits of taking time for opportunities that nurture the spirit, such as solitude, music and contemplation. Participants in the groups with which I worked certainly recognised the way in which their own exploration of spirituality benefited their health and even sanity. Personal and professional exploration of spirituality intertwined and overlapped during the life of the group. One study of health care workers suggested that they experienced beneficial spiritual growth while working in palliative care, including living more intensely and being able to enjoy the here and now (Cornette 1997, p.12). In this way, the holistic approach reaches beyond the working environment, reminding participants not to neglect their own spirituality but to remember to care for themselves, and in the long term this will help them care effectively for clients and carers.

Attending to spirituality is, then, an investment in the very essence of who we are; supporting our understanding of what gives life meaning and purpose, and how that is expressed now and in the future; it should have a positive effect on our own health and well-being. This investment has benefits for us, perhaps helping us cope with difficult aspects of our lives including issues at work but it also affects our work itself through the connections we have with colleagues and clients. Individual health care professionals who are more aware of (and more comfortable with) their own spirituality seem better able to recognise and respond to spirituality in others. If their own spirituality is healthy, for example, they will not be threatened when someone struggles to articulate a feeling that life is without meaning or expresses other causes of spiritual distress; they will be able to listen rather than block what they are hearing, and respond appropriately; this response may contribute to that person's recovery.

Learning about spirituality within the health care team suggests a practical way of responding to this tension between cost and benefit; exploring spirituality in a safe but challenging group gives participants greater confidence about the provision of spiritual care, reducing stress and encouraging self-care as well as providing support. Better understanding should ensure that spiritual care is integrated into other aspects of health care rather than becoming yet another task to add on. Enhanced personal and professional awareness of spirituality actually helps health care professionals recognise and respond to spiritual need in ways that reduce their own stress and sense of failure.

Spiritual assessment

World Health Organization (WHO) guidelines for palliative care suggest that spiritual care should include assessment of spirituality and the provision of appropriate spiritual help and support; a process that is underpinned by attentive listening and respect for individual beliefs (World Health Organization Expert Committee 1990, pp.51–2). This is more easily said than done. Again, the NICE guidelines for supportive and palliative care for adults with cancer state that the priorities for further research in spiritual support are the assessment of need and the best way of providing spiritual support (King's College London 2004, p.39). Health care professionals expect to work with clients with very different views and often need to ask about sensitive concerns – for example, related to sexuality or physical care – but spirituality remains difficult to assess in a meaningful way. A remote tick-box approach seems particularly unhelpful for such a personal and sensitive issue; ideally, spiritual assessment should not be carried out in isolation but rather should occur as an integral part of the whole health care approach. The need for any assessment to be part of a continuing process rather than a one-off opportunity is also important. A number of researchers suggest ways of assessing spirituality: Stoll's pioneering work (1979), based in America, is often quoted, but others include Highfield (1992), Narayanasamy (2004) and Post-White *et al.* (1996). While there is widespread recognition that some form of assessment would be helpful, there does not yet appear to be any agreement about the best approach, hence the suggestion from research for NICE that this is an area where significant additional work is needed (King's College London 2004, p.39).

Any assessment of spirituality needs to be underpinned by grounded reflective learning of the sort I have been describing, so that individual members of the health care team have the knowledge, skills and confidence to recognise a broad range of spiritual needs and react appropriately during the assessment process. Spirituality is an intangible and elusive concept; helpful discussions about spirituality are more likely to emerge within the context of a therapeutic relationship where there is some understanding of what spirituality is about and a recognition that assessment will not result in easy answers or tidy care plans. Clients and carers themselves may struggle to articulate their own confusion and need, and may be unaware of where to turn for spiritual support. Being alert to signs of spirituality in ourselves and others, responding positively to tangential comments or stories that seem to relate to spirituality, giving active attention to the whole person and what makes that person who they are: all these provide subtle signals that it is acceptable to talk about such intimate aspects of self. This overall attitude and approach provides a suitable setting in which to carry out more formal assessments of spirituality.

Putting assessment into practice

This understanding of spiritual assessment is reflected in the experience of the groups of health care staff that I worked with; we had spent a significant amount of time reflecting on the nature and expression of spirituality, an experience that had made us much more aware of spirituality and more comfortable talking about it with other people, including clients. Even so, we struggled as we tried to use some of the standard spiritual assessment questions available at the time; they felt wooden and intrusive and seemed to be occurring out of context. Some of our disquiet was almost certainly related to being unfamiliar with this process plus the need to reword some questions to be more appropriate for British recipients. Still we were left feeling that formal assessment could actually limit our understanding of someone's spirituality rather than enhance it. Spiritual assessment is complex for many of the same reasons that learning about spirituality is difficult; it is a deeply personal and emotive issue that is hard to talk about and carries the intrinsic risk of painful misunderstanding. Practical outward activities that express spirituality, such as religious practice, can be assessed much more easily, but to concentrate solely on these somehow misses the point. What is needed is the creation of opportunities to raise deeper concerns about meaning and purpose, hope or connection without becoming locked into a formal assessment process. Knowing from our own experience how difficult it was to start talking about these things, we wanted to ensure that clients felt able to raise and explore such personal issues if they wished. So there were clear reasons why we wanted specifically to include assessment of spirituality as a routine; we just struggled to see how to do that effectively!

After a period of experimentation, one group member described how she envisaged using a combination of questions rather than any specific assessment tool:

> I could sort of imagine starting off talking with something like 'Is it important for you to have a sense of hope?' or 'What inner resources do you draw on for hope?' Then I think I could go as far as to say 'Do you pray?', because I think that is a very generic term, which perhaps would lead on to say, you know, 'So, what sort of things do you find helpful about that?' I don't mean that then I'd necessarily explore their religious beliefs, but to say that would be [asking] what they are doing that might be facilitated by the health professional being able to talk to them about spirituality and about whether at the moment they were in touch with that side of themselves or not. Because that would be the reason for my question, not to find out whether they wanted to see the vicar, you know, but more to do with…what might happen from those conversations. It doesn't want to be automatic. The message I'm giving says 'Do you want to talk to me about that inner self that you might be turning to?' … I think that question would bring that response. And I think then the thing to ask is 'Would it help you to talk about the fact that you might not be able to draw on that part of you at the moment' or 'What might help you to draw on that more?' and 'What's sort of blocking you from being able to do that?' And I think that would be really helpful and, given that what we're trying to do is really help people express their concerns, not put the plaster over [them], I think that that would be the right opening for me.

This approach fitted into the experience of one of the health care teams with which I worked (Leedham and Platt 1998). Here a shared, multi-professional assessment tool was already being used and this allowed any member of the multi-professional team to complete an initial assessment for a new client. This assessment formed the basis of shared documentation and was added to by other members of the team during subsequent contacts. Initially, spirituality was not mentioned specifically at any stage of the assessment, although it could be raised in a general section entitled 'Other concerns'. Conscious of the difficulty of talking about this topic, the group exploring spirituality on behalf of the team suggested making this a more specific theme in the generic assessment form without setting definite assessment questions. Spirituality was simply noted as a heading in the documentation with some suggestions for areas to explore and possible phrases or questions to use. Group members tried questions from a number of different sources themselves, some of which are given in Box 6.1, eventually agreeing that while these offered possible openings they were not obligatory and it was important to use language that was understandable to clients. Spirituality could be raised as a theme at any point during the assessment process, additional notes could also be added at a later stage. Initial assessment usually occurred at an early stage of our involvement with clients (often at the first meeting) and it was felt more appropriate that discussions about spirituality would normally occur later, when a relationship has been established with a key worker, even though we recognised that this meant that spirituality could be forgotten. We recognised the need for sensitivity when asking such direct and personal questions, and the importance of explaining why such questions are being asked. Rather than a single one-off assessment, we felt spirituality should be something that could be returned to at different stages.

This approach was discussed with the wider team and eventually agreed upon as the approach to be taken. This decision was made in the clear knowledge that opportunities for continuing professional education about spirituality were available for all members of the health care team and a shared understanding of spirituality was being developed. The initial discussion group that was based within this team had worked for over a year to develop a shared understanding of spirituality; continuing professional development opportunities enabled other staff to begin to share this understanding. This common and agreed approach was essential as we worked towards a form of spiritual assessment that made sense to ourselves and our clients. Language and terminology remained a concern; spirituality will never be a word that is easily or commonly understood and anyone involved in spiritual care needs to

Box 6.1 Suggested questions for spiritual assessment

Meaning and purpose

- What are some of the things that give you a sense of purpose?
- Do you have a specific aim that is important to you at the moment?
- Do you believe in any kind of existence after this life?
- Has your illness changed your attitude to the future?
- What bothers you most about being ill?

Security and hope

- What are your sources of strength and hope?
- Who do you turn to when you need help? In what ways do they help?
- What inner resources do you draw upon?
- Where do you go for comfort or support?
- Who or what do you depend on when things go wrong?

Religion / spirituality

- Do you consider yourself to be religious or spiritual?
- How does this affect you? Has being ill changed this?
- Is prayer helpful to you? Can you talk about how?
- Is there anything we can do to support your spiritual/religious practice?

Questions adapted from Stoll 1979, pp.1574–7;
Highfield 1992, pp.3–4; Georgesen and Dungan, p.379;
Post-White *et al.* 1996, pp.1571–9

remain alert to verbal and non-verbal cues about this topic. The generic assessment tool in use at the care centre already included a number of related issues such as relationships, coping strategies and general health and well-being, but specifically including spirituality demonstrated our commitment to holistic care and ensured that clients who wished to talk about spiritual concerns were able to do so freely. Identifying spirituality in this way ensured that there was a reminder to explore spirituality with every client rather than waiting for it to be raised in a recognisable form or relying on the interests of the health care professionals involved.

Remembering the importance of the journey in the enquiry group's discussions, another possibility was to use the idea of journey as a way of asking people to talk about spirituality during their lifetime, either directly or though a journal, story or art work, as with spiritual life maps (Hodge 2005). In whatever way spirituality was explored, key issues could be documented as prompts to later discussions if needed. Having explored spiritual concerns clients may put them aside again but this would be from choice rather than lack of opportunity. Equally they may find themselves continuing to explore this area in increasing depth for the first time in their lives.

Providing spiritual care

Underlying our discussions about spiritual care was a serious question about whether it was possible to provide such care at all. Spirituality is an essentially personal and individual attribute of human beings; supporting spiritual growth or reducing spiritual distress is even harder than providing food or medication, and providing those is not always easy! The possibility that we might be able to support such a growth process flickered tantalisingly in front of us, yet we remained conscious of the dangers of 'doing spirituality' to people and of the potential cost of such work. We were no longer surprised to find that staff who are more aware of their own spirituality seem better able to recognise and respond to spiritual concerns in others (see, for example, Waugh 1992, p.227; Ross 1997a, p.41). We could see how as our own awareness of spirituality had increased, we had become more confident when talking to people about this issue. Not that we felt we had all the answers but we were no longer so worried by our incomplete knowledge, recognising how much more there would always be to learn. We hoped that this would, at the very least, help us avoid accidentally crushing clients who wished to explore spirituality for themselves. Basic skills, such as being a good listener, showing empathy and being available to others, all supported the provision of spiritual care and we could see how practical activities such as complementary therapies, opportunities for relaxation or diversion also made a contribution. The personal human contribution of attributes such as compassion and acceptance were also vitally important. All these things had existed before we began to explore spirituality; what was new was our acceptance of the spiritual dimension as an integral part of health care that was relevant to everyone. This broad acceptance was no longer simply an interesting theoretical idea but something in which we were involved, that affected us personally as well as in our professional work. Our eyes had been opened and we now saw life differently because of that change in understanding.

This sort of experience suggests that an important factor in the nurture of spirituality is the encouragement and freedom to explore spirituality. Again and again the groups I worked with returned to the idea of the journey as a metaphor for spirituality; the sense of search, sometimes of struggle, to reach understanding about what spirituality was and how it affected people was potent. The understanding that spirituality was linked to an individual's search for meaning, purpose or hope reinforced this view. For us this search did not have an uncomfortable sense of striving, although we saw that it could do, but rather the fascination of a subject where there always seemed more to explore and that was pertinent to so much of life. In the palliative care centre where many of those involved worked, clients were generally physically well enough to explore these concerns, although life-threatening illness had provided an important catalyst for spiritual exploration. We did see how at the very end of life spiritual needs may change, particularly where the client is slipping into unconsciousness. A broader understanding of spirituality, as described previously, is linked to a wider provision of spiritual support that makes it clear that there are different ways to express and nurture spirituality. We had found our differences illuminating and were keen that individuals using the centre should also have that freedom to explore spirituality in different ways without feeling that there is one simple answer. Spiritual care should always be underpinned by respect for human life and dignity even when people have very different ideas from our own.

A safe place to be

At the heart of spiritual care, just as in learning about spirituality, is the provision of a safe space where the spiritual dimension can be recognised and valued, although it might also be challenged. In this space, spirituality can be discussed openly by those clients who wish to do so, knowing that their views will be heard and respected without fear of misinterpretation or stigma. Differing ideas about spirituality can be recognised and respected without embarrassment or disdain, creating a context where people can discuss their spirituality openly, perhaps for the first time, if they wish to do so. Of course spiritual care is not only about talk and discussion but other aspects of spiritual support became better recognised and accepted where there was a shared understanding of spirituality. The time spent developing a shared understanding and approach to spirituality meant that we could see the spiritual dimension lived out in a variety of practical activities. For us, the experience of developing a space in which to explore spirituality freely, while retaining both the challenge and support of other people, had been a key element in nurturing spirituality and we wanted this to be available to others as well. Continuing professional education opportunities offering a safe space where health care teams could reflect on spirituality together, integrating the personal and professional domains, provided an essential foundation for the provision of spiritual care. Without this process, it was hard to see how actual spiritual care could be provided in a sustained and consistent way.

7

Outcomes and Opportunities

Learning affecting practice

Growing interest in alternative and complementary therapies has highlighted the importance of gathering evidence about all such therapeutic interventions; it also demonstrates the difficulty of doing so. Spiritual care also needs to be gathering evidence about the effectiveness of differing aspects of practice; indeed, such evidence is beginning to be gathered as is demonstrated by its inclusion in the NICE guidelines on palliative and supportive care for adults with cancer (National Institute for Clinical Excellence 2004). If spirituality is as important as I have suggested, then it should be considered just as carefully as any other intervention, and questions about process and outcomes should be asked in the same way as for any other aspect of health care. To challenge ideas about spirituality and holistic care is helpful, indicating greater respect for those ideas than either blind acceptance or simple disregard. Challenge, as in our discussion groups, assumes that the ideas of spirituality are valid and therefore open to greater understanding. On this basis differing approaches can be explored because there are things to learn, not just to be disproved. Developing an evidence-based approach to spirituality and spiritual care is difficult when the strict criteria of medical science, as in the randomised control trial, exclude much that would be helpful in exploring spirituality. Critics of traditional research methods, such as Reason and Rowan (1981) or Reason and Heron (1985), call for a different methodology that will provide better evidence about this particular aspect of health care. We have already seen how human spirituality and spiritual care is difficult to understand and practise, so it should surely come as no surprise that it is difficult to research even when there is the will to do so. If spirituality is so integral an element of each human being, the effect of attending to it will be spread widely throughout health care; not all these effects will be visible or open to direct measurement. Exploring spirituality with others and the effect of this on spiritual care, as we have discussed, is one opportunity to develop a better understanding. This was the purpose of the groups with which I worked and some of the outcomes of that process are explored in this chapter.

Think for a moment about the impact of understanding spirituality in the way we have been considering. Spirituality affects individual health care staff in their personal and professional lives; it affects their outlook on life and the choices they make; their own health and well-being as well as the work they do and the people they connect with through that work. It may mean that they work in different ways or with a different perspective. Becoming more aware of spirituality in this way may be uncomfortable or even painful, even if it is clearly beneficial. Ultimately this process should bear fruit in people's lives, including, for example, greater personal awareness about their own sense of meaning and purpose, or working in ways that feel more connected and holistic. The outcome of being more aware of spirituality, both personally and professionally, will be wide-reaching, subtle and certainly not easy to quantify.

As well as considering the outcomes of the holistic approach, with particular reference to spirituality, we need to look at how to enable people to work in this way. There are different ways of encouraging a more holistic approach and of increasing awareness of spirituality and providing effective spiritual care. This book has advocated reflective learning, particularly in the context of multi-professional health care teams, to integrate ideas about spirituality into actual practice. My experience of exploring spirituality with groups of staff and volunteers in this way has been positive but that is not, of course, the only approach and it does have a cost in terms of time and commitment, as well as the risk of damaging the team if it all goes horribly wrong. From the outset, our specific aim in each of the groups was to 'explore our own spirituality with a view to how that informs our work', something that we did achieve. We considered that the outcomes of this process should be reflected in our working practices as well as our personal lives; part of our shared exploration was about making spiritual care a reality rather than mere rhetoric. Again this was achieved with changes to our practice, some of which are explored below, emerging from our recognition that the spiritual domain is integral to each human being. Multi-professional team members electing to explore spirituality in the ways this book suggests should similarly expect to see changes in their personal and professional lives, changes that relate to the team as a whole as well as to individual members. Measuring those changes is complex and requires a rather different approach to research and audit than is commonly used in health services.

Outcomes of exploring spirituality

The process of exploring spirituality with others led to unexpected personal and professional changes as we began to engage with both the topic and the group itself. Vague talk about spirituality, experiences with clients or colleagues and the occasional reference in a conference or journal became more focused as we established a framework within which to understand this complex subject and developed a safe place in which to explore it. Although the personal and professional outcomes of this process were intertwined, I have separated them here for practical reasons.

Time spent by teams or organisations exploring spirituality should have positive outcomes that affect the organisation as well as benefitting the individuals who take part. The exploratory groups I worked with occurred in the context of health care teams; health care provided the context and impetus for our shared exploration and we expected it to have work-related outcomes. Although we recognised from the beginning that personal and professional aspects of spirituality were intertwined, I was initially surprised at the extent to which some individuals used the group to explore their personal spirituality. With hindsight, these were probably individuals for whom exploring spirituality in this way was quite a new experience. In the longest-running group, we noted how personal exploration dominated the initial sessions and appeared to be linked to developing trust within the group as well as the need for personal development. Later we moved on to explore specific work-related issues, such as assessment and the provision of spiritual care, but this aspect clearly emerged from this initial shared foundation (see Figure 4.1 on p.67). This sense of progression was also apparent in groups with a shorter time span and clearer syllabus, although it was less marked.

Personal outcomes

We have already discussed at length the way in which spirituality has become a pervading topic within our culture. There are frequent and varied references to it in the media, advertising and the Arts, as well as more specific references in health care. What is so often missing in all this discussion is the opportunity to explore the significance and meaning of these references, particularly in ways that require a degree of challenge and discernment. Health care practice and the relevance of spirituality within it is one particular area where this process is needed, although others include education, the Arts and business. Such opportunities provide an alternative to either absorbing the current contradictory mixture wholesale or simply ignoring it, neither of which seems quite the right response. What is required is an opportunity for individuals to reflect on such references in the world where they live and work – to consider them carefully, testing them against real experience and theoretical ideas in their personal as well as professional lives. I am not suggesting that every chance encounter should be an opportunity for health care staff or their clients to stop and consider its deepest spiritual significance; this would surely become tedious and artificial, quite apart from the huge demands on time. Rather, I believe, there will be real benefits for individuals who devote time to exploring this pervasive theme with respect to their health care practice. Making time to consider my response to a relevant encounter with a patient is an opportunity for my personal and professional development in this area, with the links to my own spirituality readily apparent. I am aware in my own practice how easy it is for such encounters to slip by without learning anything from them, yet the uncomfortable questions raised by such an encounter leave their mark. How much better to be able to consider spiritual aspects of a particular critical incident in conjunction with practical and cognitive aspects and learn from them all.

Exploring those questions or concerns with other people, although challenging, provides a forum to explore my own spirituality and a group setting may help such an exploration although it is not essential. Of course, work offers only one particular opportunity to explore spirituality but the groups with which I was involved suggested it was a significant one. Even those who already felt they had a clear understanding of their own spirituality valued the opportunity to broaden their individual and personal understanding in these encounters with others and with specific reference to their work.

The experience of exploring spirituality with groups of health care staff, as I have described here, suggests that there are benefits in sharing this process, not only because it makes it happen but also because of the greater impact and opportunities it provides. All of those involved felt clearer about the whole topic of spirituality, what it was and was not, as well as how it might affect our work. This sense of greater clarity and the simple experience of discussing our ideas about spirituality with other people inspired a greater confidence in those who had been involved. Spirituality was no longer taboo, something to avoid or stumble over when it was referred to at work or by our friends and family. This confidence and clarity was very far from a sense that we now had spirituality neatly sewn up but rather that we were now more at ease with our own uncertainty and this left open the possibility of continuing to explore this area. It no longer seemed as if everyone else knew what they were talking about and we were somehow missing something. We recognised in a new and more relaxed way that spirituality was an area where our ideas and thinking would naturally change and grow as part of our human development. Individuals within the groups spoke of feeling more comfortable with the topic and with their own questions, reflecting their previous discomfort about an area where they felt clumsy and uncertain. This greater confidence meant that we were less likely to block references to spirituality or religion when other people raised the topic. One participant described how she found herself talking about spirituality with her own family for an unusually long time; another reported how the work-based group had prompted her to begin a personal exploration of a topic she would have avoided in other contexts:

> I've felt much more sparked as I've come away from [the group], I feel like I've got more energy and I know that I've been sort of talking about it and thinking things though more outside of it ... I think it's been a really valuable experience and I suppose the sentiment of saying that I think other people should have the opportunity to do it does reflect how valuable I've found it and would never, never, unless it was in this setting, have approached it.

Exploring with others added significantly to this process for the individuals who took part. Exploring spirituality is always challenging; exploring with others added to that challenge but there was also an increasing sense of support and understanding about a struggle we shared. Somehow it helped that even those who seemed confident or clear didn't have all the answers, thus opening the way to exploring further together. As we talked, it became clearer that spirituality was both highly individual and personal but also universal and communal:

> [People] should be able to think and reach their own potential as unique human beings without rules and behaviour but at the same time should have a sense of community and sharing and caring.

Exploring spirituality with other people certainly helped create the sense of shared community that was such an important part of our experience. The group developed a sense of mutual support that had benefits beyond the immediate exploration of spirituality, benefits for the team (which will be explored later) and for individuals. Of course, there was the added benefit of other people providing additional resources, more ideas and experiences, plus the fascination of seeing how our ideas were shared and where we differed. The need to articulate our ideas so that others could understand them was a huge challenge – at times frustrating, as already discussed – but that very process helped us work through some of that inarticulacy to find a language we could use to talk about spirituality. We wondered together at the way our ideas seemed to resist being captured or pinned down, seeping through our minds like smoke as we explored; as one aspect of spirituality became clearer, we began to see the incompleteness of this view and other ideas or perspectives emerged. In some sense we were always going back to the drawing board but all the time our thinking became deeper and richer with a strong and exciting sense that this would be a continuing exploration. When we heard clients struggling with these issues we did not expect to have answers, but were more able to listen and support them because of our own exploration.

Several people spoke about how exploring together acted as a catalyst for further exploration outside the group, some of which led to action or personal changes, some very small, others larger, but all part of a continuing process in which the group simply played a part. Taking time to focus on spirituality and explore it in an open and questioning environment was an important element of this process; individuals described how they had been prompted to explore their personal spirituality in new ways, as these examples suggest:

> I've come to the point where for the first time ever I have considered actively seeking a group to share some of my feelings and thoughts about spirituality. [That's come from] having the freedom to explore and to dabble and just be interested in it for its own sake.

> I've tended to come from this angle that I was very much a failed Christian and very doubting but I've come to a point where I'm more OK with that. I'm not actually on the outside of Christianity any more, I'm within it but, because of the nature of my mind, I'll always be questioning...and the doubts are OK to have. That's quite a movement for me and feels like I have roots and a place to start from.

Professional or work-related outcomes

The groups that I worked with encouraged individuals to explore spirituality specifically in terms of their working or professional practice. Individually and together we reflected on critical incidents or other experiences that had raised questions or highlighted concerns about spirituality, recognising that such 'teachable moments' (Karpiak 1992, p.53) had helped shape our understanding of spirituality. Many of the positive outcomes for individuals already discussed have additional benefits for professional practice as well as people's personal lives. A clear focus on spirituality ensured that individuals were far more aware of the whole issue in their work, more attuned to any references to spirituality in discussions with clients and colleagues:

> I haven't come up with any answers as to what [spirituality] is and how we should be doing it … I don't think I expected to. The positive side still feels very much that it's on my agenda because of doing this group so I'm aware of it and developing in that sense.

Greater understanding of the whole concept of spirituality, including a sense of the breadth of ideas involved, helped. Participants were more able to recognise when these issues were being raised, sometimes rather diffidently or tangentially, by clients or colleagues. Increased awareness, coupled with greater confidence, ensured that health care professionals could respond positively to clients rather than blocking any references to spirituality.

Recognising our own inarticulacy and confusion helped us understand how others might be feeling as they started to think and talk about spirituality. The need to articulate our ideas for other people, sometimes with very different viewpoints, had prompted us to explore this issue more widely and deeply in order to find words and images that other people could understand. Again, instead of shying away from discussions about spirituality, we were willing to struggle to find words, as this example illustrates:

> I don't normally get involved in discussions about religion as a separate thing but I saw a girl last week for whom religion had previously been a coping strategy and very helpful for her. I wanted to explore this but I couldn't think of the words; I didn't know how to phrase the question to ask about it in the right words. I came up with a real sort of grammatical problem because it was very, very unfamiliar to me. I didn't know whether I was trivialising it, offending her or hitting it right. It was like talking in a different language. I was just going along and started the sentence and she finished it off and it was OK. I think it was, on a very practical level, quite helpful to have had that discussion.

Another participant described how the group had provided a sounding board when spiritual issues were raised within her work with clients:

> It feels good to have somewhere to bring it back, to bring those issues back and explore that within the group and that increases my confidence to go out and tackle those issues again.

In all the groups we found that encounters with each other increased our confidence to raise spirituality as an issue in encounters with clients, particularly as our ideas developed. Whether spirituality was explored further depended on what the client wanted, rather than on what the health care professional was willing to allow.

Multi-professional team or group outcomes

One of the groups I worked with had the added advantage of being given a remit to consider this issue on behalf of the whole multi-professional team (of which they formed a significant part). This meant that, as we explored spirituality together, we were able to develop and agree a framework that could then be shared by the whole team. This framework helped ensure greater consistency, particularly in assessment and care, but it also gave members of the team greater confidence. They knew that in this personal, and sometimes difficult, subject they were not acting as isolated individuals but as part of a team with a shared understanding and approach. The process of working together to reach agreement helped refine and shape our ideas, creating something for the team that was greater than our individual ideas. This understanding continued to be refined over time as we worked with it and began to incorporate these ideas into different areas of our practice. Later, the wider team also began to reflect on our ideas and further development occurred. Spirituality became a more explicit element within our service, with greater openness about what that meant and a clear recognition that it affected all areas of service provision. The two main outcomes for this group were to include spirituality in the care centre's assessment tools and to develop a training module about spirituality for use with other staff and volunteers, both of which have been discussed in earlier chapters. Individual members of the group also worked to ensure spirituality was included in the continuing review of other activities within the centre, including the physical environment, practical activities and complementary therapies.

As more opportunities to explore spirituality were offered to the team, this shared understanding provided a base from which other staff, including those who were new, could explore spirituality for themselves. For example, discussions about the links and differences between religion and spirituality made us more aware of how we might impose, even unconsciously, our own beliefs and values; agreement that spirituality is part of every human being encouraged us to explore spiritual needs more openly; experiencing the variety of actual religious practice in discussions with others broke open stereotypical ideas about different faith groups. Greater recognition of the place of spirituality in health care not only made for some interesting and helpful conversations with clients and colleagues, it also helped develop a level of competence in this area of health care. We have already explored the need for education about spirituality among health care staff of all grades and professions; educational groups, such as the ones I have been describing, provide ideal opportunities for individuals to explore spirituality quite practically, yet in some depth, with other health care professionals working in similar situations. Over time, these experiences build up a level of practical expertise and confidence about this subject that has a significant effect on practice.

The opportunity to explore this topic together also appeared to affect working relationships in the group and the team as a whole, building connections with each other as well as shared knowledge. Exploring an element of ourselves that was so personal, including some stormy discussions, drew us closer although we recognised that it could have had the opposite effect. Inevitably we understood more about our fellow group members and that put a different dimension into working relationships. Indeed the experience left us curious to understand how other people within the team felt about spirituality, what their ideas were and what had shaped those beliefs. There was a sense of connection within the group that appeared to stem from sharing this personal dimension of ourselves and this helped create a sense of team cohesion. Perhaps this is partly because spirituality is so rarely talked about, but I sense it is also because the very subject of spirituality requires a degree of personal openness and vulnerability. Of course, that inevitably means there is a risk of frustration and discomfort when teams explore spirituality together, particularly where contradictory beliefs are strongly held. The whole group must recognise this and be committed to working together to find a way through such difficulties, including adherence to clear ground rules, as outlined in an earlier chapter. The decision to explore spirituality as a team should not be taken lightly, demanding as it does a level of personal and professional commitment to the process that goes beyond simply the time required. Having made that clear, my experience suggests that when health care teams do manage to overcome the usual barriers to talking about spirituality they will find the experience affirms and strengthens the bonds between them.

One of the concerns expressed was that those not involved in exploring spirituality would feel excluded from future discussions and operational outcomes. Some people in our health care team clearly felt excluded by the very topic, while others were excluded by practical issues of timing or availability.

Far from building team cohesion this could easily have had the negative effect of creating division and dissent, perhaps even aggravating existing divisions within the team – for example, between different staff groups. In order to overcome this possible negative outcome, we agreed to report back to the whole team at regular intervals; this included several discussions about the purpose of the group and the nature of spirituality, plus regular feedback from the group in whole-team meetings. Later, a display outlining the purpose of the group and its initial outcomes was also made available for clients and wider members of the team. None of these things was the same as actually taking part but all appeared to go some way to avoid excluding people.

Perhaps more important was the greater openness of group members to talk about spirituality in an informal way outside of the group. Their increased confidence and interest in this area meant they were more aware of spirituality in their everyday practice and more likely to comment on or explore relevant issues with other team members. Personal information disclosed within the group was, of course, confidential but that did not mean all our discussions were secret. Indeed, participants were encouraged to test out new ideas about spirituality in the context of their everyday work and feed the results, including discussions within the wider team, back to the group. This created a great deal of interest in the topic and process, and there was a lot of interest when further opportunities for other people to explore spirituality were offered.

Changes in working practice

One important outcome of exploring spirituality was that it became quite clear that this was not just another task to add to our normal practice, neither was it an extra service for which someone should be referred to a spiritual expert such as the chaplain. Rather it was now obvious that spirituality was an integral and essential part of all health care practice almost whether we liked it or not; even attempts to ignore spirituality conveyed a message to clients. Individuals who had explored spirituality in this way, in all the groups with which I was involved, described how a better understanding of spirituality led to greater awareness, affecting our attitudes, understanding and skills. Increased awareness meant that we were more likely to recognise spiritual issues in discussions with clients or carers, and were more confident about responding when that happened. We understood that our responses would be very varied, depending on the needs of the situation and the client or carer; they might be simply to recognise and respect someone as a spiritual being, to listen as someone explored his or her own spiritual history or ideas, or to refer for more specific support to other team members, including the chaplaincy. Far from spirituality becoming simply another box to be ticked, we saw it as an underpinning element across all our practice. In particular, we explored the way in which spirituality had become a more general part of our practice with all clients, rather than something we considered only in desperation or as a last resort.

This change of approach has implications for those of us working in palliative care but also more widely. For example, the broader awareness of spirituality encouraged the team to consider spirituality as part of our overall activity, affecting everything from buildings and systems to choice of activities and therapies. We were fortunate to have access to a range of therapeutic interventions including complementary therapies and creative activities such as creative writing, art, music and gardening. We now saw how these could support spiritual as well as physical care as they offered opportunities for creativity and relaxation. Understanding that the services we offered fed the spirit as well as the mind and body became part of our regular review of activities. We also spent time considering the physical environment in which we worked, looking at use of the Arts and the need to preserve space for privacy or quiet reflection, although what we could do was limited. All this highlighted the difficulty of meeting varied needs: what counts as uplifting art or music for one person does not count as uplifting for all. We wanted to avoid simply creating a bland environment that helps no one, and to aim for something which ensures that spirituality pervades the working environment. This may include the creation or use of a sacred space (perhaps a chapel or prayer room) as well as wider consideration of the physical environment including use of plants and decor, access to the outdoors and art work. One positive outcome of our discussions was that we were now able to talk these ideas through as a team with a shared understanding of spirituality; this made for more ideas and better decisions.

There is no doubt that activity in the care centre changed as a result of the inquiry into spirituality, but whether this more holistic understanding was sustained remains open to question. I suspect it will be a continuing effort to ensure spirituality is not squeezed out by other seemingly urgent or practical matters. Spirituality sometimes seems rather self-effacing, and changes in staffing or organisational demands tend to push it back into obscurity. Continued attention will be required to ensure that it remains an integral part of health care practice. For these reasons, continuing professional development related to spirituality is essential to sustain understanding and competence in this area. Any attempt to explore the theme of spirituality without understanding both its personal and professional implications is likely to be uncomfortable and painful for both staff and clients. Similarly, I suspect that attempts to impose a policy about spirituality and spiritual care without a shared exploration such as we have described are doomed to failure.

Health-related outcomes

Discussions of outcomes have, so far, focused mostly on those related to knowledge and understanding of spirituality. Yet if the spiritual dimension is central to being human, it is not unreasonable to think that attending to the health of the spirit should affect total health and well-being (body, mind and spirit), as suggested in Chapter 5. The values and beliefs that are such a central part of spirituality affect the decisions we all make about life, even though that effect is sometimes hidden or unconscious. Decisions about diet and lifestyle, relationships or work are affected, for example, by the value we give to ourselves and other people, and will have a huge influence on our health and well-being. Of course, the values we have and the choices we make are in turn affected by many things, including culture, upbringing and resources. Similarly, health and well-being are influenced by many factors that are outside our control and not a matter of choice. Who would choose to experience any life-threatening disease? Yet how we respond to that disease is affected by our beliefs and values. Our tolerance of pain or stress, our sense of self-worth and the strength of our personal support networks – all these affect how we cope with disease or difficulty. Health care professionals need to recognise and value such connections if they are to support their clients in a holistic way, recognising the complexity of people's lives rather than just the presenting symptoms or particular diagnoses. It is not for the health care team to resolve that complexity, but understanding it (to a degree) may help us work more effectively with clients. The experiences described in this book lead me to suggest that a better understanding of spirituality can help us do just that.

There is, though, a further argument that goes beyond this to suggest that the health of an individual's spirit affects the health of his or her mind and body. Certainly loss of hope, a sense of meaninglessness or the inability to connect with others are seen as aspects of ill health, so perhaps the opposite is also true and individuals who attend to their spirit (for example, who have a clear sense of purpose in life or strong relationships with others) are either less likely to be ill or will cope better with the effects of illness. Such a link should not be made too simplistically but, if we believe in the holistic nature of human beings, it makes sense that the health of body, mind and spirit are closely interconnected. This is a further reminder that spirituality is not just an added luxury but an integral element of the health care team's work, influencing the well-being of all those involved, clients, carers or, indeed, health care staff themselves.

In this context, some researchers are looking at the links between spirituality and health. Simplistically such ideas generate headlines such as 'psalms and sermons could save you' (Illman 1998) or 'meditation leads to longer life' (Adam 2005), but this risks trivialising the complex issues involved. Some of the positive links between religious practice and health can be explained by social benefits, such as a supportive community, or by lifestyle choices, such as the restriction of alcohol or smoking, but the overall relationship appears to be more complex. Religious practices (such as lifestyle or church attendance) are easier to measure than more metaphysical aspects of religion or spirituality and these appear to have some health benefits. Some researchers claim that there are also positive links between religion and health that are unrelated to social or behavioural choices. For example, in America, the National Institute for Health Care Research, a privately funded non-profit-making advocacy organisation, has published extensive literature reviews suggesting that religious faith and practice can be positively linked to health status (Levin, Larson and Puchalski 1997; Ziegler 1998). Other writers (such as Benson with Stark 1996; Burne 2000, 2004) also highlight the links between personality and health. Some of this evidence is disputed (Sloan, Bagiella and Powell 1999) and a clearer distinction between spirituality and religion in such research would be helpful. It is surely beneficial that organisations such as NICE and the Cochrane Centre are paying some attention to spirituality and religion, demonstrating that this is an aspect of health to be considered thoughtfully rather than simply dismissed. Much more research is certainly needed but evidence does seem to be growing that religion and spirituality, in differing ways, can be linked to positive physical and mental well-being (King's College London 2004; NICE 2004; Speck, Higginson and Addington-Hall 2004). That alone suggests health care professionals should not ignore this aspect of their clients' care if not their own health.

A number of themes can be seen in the links between religion or spirituality and well-being that extend beyond the lifestyle choices outlined earlier. For example, there appear to be health benefits connected to involvement in a faith community. These may be linked to religious practices, such as prayer or meditation, or strong social networks. The support of a faith community may have a positive effect on coping with illness and mental health. Another emerging theme deals with the links, both positive and negative, between personality and health. While negative emotions, such as anger or depression, appear to increase the risk of disease, the opposite also appears to be true. Positive emotions, such as happiness or optimism, support the body's own defence against disease. This is analogous to the idea that complementary therapies strengthen the body's own defence against disease. The effect of personality and emotions on health outcomes appears to work through the nervous system and immune response. An angry or unhappy individual is more susceptible, for example, to higher blood pressure and increased levels of homocysteine, both linked to heart disease. Of course, recognising links between personality and health does not immediately lead to better health, although it may explain why some people are healthier than others. Neither is this a matter of simply telling people to cheer up and be healthy, rather understanding these links opens up new possibilities for promoting health – for example, using cognitive behavioural therapy to develop positive responses to stressful situations or encouraging faith communities to build links with mental health service users.

Not unconnected with these ideas is the sense that spirituality may have a positive effect on health by supporting a more balanced lifestyle. Greater awareness of their spirituality is a first step towards ensuring individuals nurture their spirit as well as the body and mind. People will do that in many different ways but spirituality reminds us that there is more to life than meeting our basic need for food and shelter. Activities such as music, creativity in writing, art or even cooking, walking in the countryside, all feed that part of us that searches restlessly for the transcendent. Similarly the human instinct for love reaches out beyond the self in acts of altruism, as described by the Archbishop of Canterbury at an act of remembrance for the victims of the 2004 tsunami in the Indian Ocean:

> The human response to pain and tragedy is as unreasonable as so much of the tragedy itself. It is generous and creative, self forgetful, capable of doing what sometimes seem very small or ineffectual things simply because they are worth doing for the sake of honouring other human beings ... Despite all the ways we train ourselves out of it by selfishness and busyness, love is essentially the most natural thing for us. (Rowan Williams, quoted in *Church Times* 2005, p.3)

I would suggest that this instinct for transcendence is part of spiritual awareness, promoting health by reminding human beings what is important. Remembering the spiritual creates a sense of perspective and an awareness of the wider context beyond our own concerns. Specific activities, such as meditation, can be a far more effective response to stressful situations than potentially damaging or addictive behaviours. Opportunities to relax, for example, through walking in the countryside or, again, through meditation or prayer, also bring long-term benefits for physical and mental health. Having a sense of meaning and purpose about life, a strong connection with other people and with the wider world, as well as a positive hope for the future, all aspects of spirituality that we have described, are likely to have a positive effect on total health and well-being in myriad ways. Becoming more aware of spirituality is only the first step towards making health-promoting decisions but that first step is important.

The understanding that spirituality can promote positive health is also relevant in the treatment of existing disease. Spiritual care might lead to a reduction in the length of hospital stays, lower levels of medication or even decreased admissions. By reducing anxiety or loss of purpose, spirituality can lead to relaxation that enhances the body's healing ability as well as helping individuals cope with their disease and its treatment. This is recognised, for example, in strong positive evidence for the beneficial effect of therapies, such as relaxation, in reducing the negative side effects of treatment as well as limited evidence that quality of life and other functional outcomes are better (NICE 2002, p.30). I know from my own limited experience that stress and anxiety make pain feel more acute and hard to bear. The support of my family and friends, knowing that I am not alone as well as an awareness (admittedly sometimes hard to hold on to) that life is more than the pain I am feeling, all help reduce my distress.

A shared holistic approach to health care, including an understanding of spirituality, will promote health and healing. Of course, healing does not mean cure – an individual may remain chronically ill yet still experience a sense of healing linked to reduced pain, forgiveness or restored relationships. Health care teams that are comfortable with these broader aspects of health care will demonstrate an acceptance of the whole person and a willingness to talk about spiritual issues such as meaning or hope in parallel with other aspects of disease and treatment. Two NICE reports (2002, 2004) note that the ability of health care professionals to provide the spiritual and social support that clients need is currently very limited. Again, I suspect that health care teams who take the issue of spirituality and spiritual care seriously will find they are better equipped to support clients in a number of ways. More comfortable with difficult questions, more willing to listen without having an answer and more accepting of people as whole human beings.

Developing validity in spirituality

The emphasis on evidence-based medicine makes spiritual care vulnerable without a strong research base. It is certainly possible to suggest that spirituality can have positive effects on health, as I have done, but such positive effects do not necessarily mean either avoiding illness or an automatic cure. An individual's response to a disease and treatments is hugely variable and still something of a mystery. The human spirit, whatever that is, can be expected to affect health and well-being, but understanding quite how that happens and measuring the effect is far from easy. Outcome measures, such as morbidity and mortality, provide only limited quantitative data about the effectiveness of this holistic approach. How, for example, can such measurements illuminate the experience of the client who dies at peace because he or she had the opportunity to reflect on his or her life and find in it a sense of meaning and purpose?

There is now a growing body of research data about spirituality in the UK. A variety of quantitative and qualitative methods are being used to gather information about spirituality in different areas of health care from the perspective of both clients and staff. Some examples of such research are noted below, and many have been referred to already in other parts of this book. Evidence for the NICE report on supportive and palliative care for adults with cancer (King's College London 2004) summarises the specific (but limited) evidence about spiritual care for this area of practice, noting the need for further study. An example of a study looking at the client's view of spirituality is the work by Simsen (1985), who carried out a descriptive study with patients in hospital using a mixture of semi-structured and in-depth interviews. She identified the importance of meaning in the spirituality of patients in hospital (this work was referred to in Chapter 5). Two key examples of research involving health care staff are Waugh's descriptive study (1992) using questionnaires and some interviews to explore the perceptions of nursing staff on elderly care wards about spirituality and spiritual care, plus McSherry's (1997) descriptive study using a questionnaire to identify perceptions of spirituality among nursing staff throughout a large NHS trust. Both studies have been referred to elsewhere (for example, in Chapter 3). There is clearly a need for further research on all aspects of spirituality and spiritual care in the context of health care. As this body of evidence grows there will also be a need for further reviews and meta-analyses in different areas of health care. It is essential for anyone interested in this topic to be aware that new evidence is becoming available all the time as interest grows.

Spirituality is essentially about an indefinable quality of the human spirit, the art of living and dying, of relationships and wholeness. It seems of little value, even if it were possible, to neatly package such issues for a randomised control trial. Even if such a trial were envisaged, the results obtained would surely tell us little of value about the nature of spirituality. Thankfully, qualitative approaches to research are becoming more acceptable in health care and offer greater possibilities in an area such as spirituality. The emphasis on wholeness in spirituality supports the need for a more participatory approach taking seriously the knowledge of all those involved and moving away from a view of research that separates the subject of the research from the neutral researcher or observer. Personal experience becomes central to this approach, viewed not as a contaminant but a resource; the challenge is to understand that experience better in the light of the ideas and experience of others, including theoretical perspectives and written material. In my own study, for example, I was part of the group being researched; my own beliefs and values were open to question and debate as much as other people's, contributing to the debate rather than hidden or ignored. This approach to research requires not just a different system of measurement but an entirely different approach, where there is space to unravel ideas we usually take for granted and an acceptance of intuitive insights as well as so-called hard facts. At the end of this process there is unlikely to be a single neat answer but instead a better understanding of a complex issue and a sense of wonder as we recognise all that we still do not know. A number of qualitative research methods, such as narrative research, human inquiry and grounded theory, provide avenues through which to develop this complex web of understanding about spirituality and spiritual care.

My research into learning and spirituality, for example, used a methodology called co-operative inquiry that links periods of reflection and action in order to draw on the resources of all those involved in the research. Like other forms of human inquiry (Reason and Rowan 1981), this approach aims to be *objectively subjective*, integrating theory and practice to create new understanding that is rooted in actual experience yet still systematic and rigorous in its development. Reflective cycles built into the research process ensure that periods of shared group reflection alternate with periods of activity (see Figure 7.1). This approach enabled us to test out our new and developing ideas against practical experience at work, bringing what we discovered to the group for further reflection and learning. For example, in the second reflective phase, the group agreed to focus on spiritual care and assessment. After quite a lot of discussion about this theme in the whole group, two participants elected to work on spiritual assessment in the second action phase. This included contacting other palliative care centres to find out what assessment tools were used there, trying out different spirituality assessments in their own work and being more aware of spirituality within their normal work. The results of this activity were brought back to the whole group for further reflection.

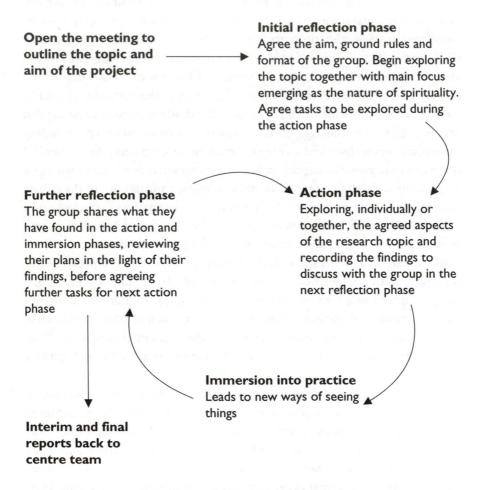

Open the meeting to outline the topic and aim of the project

Initial reflection phase
Agree the aim, ground rules and format of the group. Begin exploring the topic together with main focus emerging as the nature of spirituality. Agree tasks to be explored during the action phase

Further reflection phase
The group shares what they have found in the action and immersion phases, reviewing their plans in the light of their findings, before agreeing further tasks for next action phase

Action phase
Exploring, individually or together, the agreed aspects of the research topic and recording the findings to discuss with the group in the next reflection phase

Immersion into practice
Leads to new ways of seeing things

Interim and final reports back to centre team

Figure 7.1 The co-operative inquiry cycle (based on Heron 1996)

Qualitative data can demonstrate helpfully the subtle effect of spirituality within health care, and lead to increased understanding of this complex and very human subject. Yet stereotyping quantitative research methodologies as bad and qualitative methods as good, or vice versa, is too simplistic; both have value in health care research even in an area such as spirituality. Quantitative data on health outcomes has been reported, for example, in connection with the effect of both intercessory prayer (*Bandolier* 1997) or meditation (Canter and Ernst 2004); such data contribute to the debate but give only a small part of the picture and need to be interpreted carefully. Clients who are ill do not exist in laboratory conditions; symptom control, supportive care, human respect, physical and social environment, as well as the client's own beliefs and values, all play a part in their experience and affect the outcome of any treatment. Some, or even all, of these things may, or may not, be specifically linked to religion and spirituality in the minds of both staff and client. There are a great many variables to be considered and interpreting quantitative data is never going to be easy. Yet such quantitative data is responding to questions about effectiveness and benefit that clients are increasingly asking about all aspects of health care; interpreting any such data is never going to be easy.

Holistic care is a whole approach, including a wide spectrum of activities and treatments, and underpinned by a particular attitude that is understanding of human nature. Clients say they want to be treated holistically, meaning that they want to be recognised and respected as whole human beings. Health care professionals want to work holistically, although that can be a struggle, with large workloads and entrenched attitudes. It would help us all to know that working holistically will make a difference to patient outcome; but researchers need to question what counts as making a difference and how we measure that difference accurately. Scientific data on health, including outcomes, is part of the answer but not the whole. A healthy scepticism and an open, enquiring mind will be of great value to health care teams that elect to explore spirituality but more than scientific knowledge will be required. A sense of wonder, a willingness to listen with respect if not agreement, and a human acknowledgement of our limitations are also needed to gain insight and understanding. This takes us back to questions about meaning and purpose, the nature of spirituality and other metaphysical questions, back to the art of health care practice and a challenge to think more about the nature of research in health care.

Standards and audit in spirituality

Throughout health care the emphasis on working to agreed standards and guidelines is supported by audit of actual practice and outcomes. The difficulties inherent in measuring the effectiveness of spiritual care, referred to above, have prevented too close an examination of this aspect of health care. Department of Health guidelines for good practice in chaplaincy do exist (2003a) and are intended to promote a flexible response to the spiritual and religious needs of all staff, patients and carers. Similarly, the Northern and Yorkshire Chaplains and Pastoral Care Committee published standards that include the provision of chaplaincy as well as level and type of service (NHS Executive Northern and Yorkshire Chaplains and Pastoral Care Committee 1995). Audit of spiritual care becomes possible when it focuses on activities such as documentation, access (for example, to a suitable worship space or faith community adviser) and assessment (Catterall *et al.* 1998). These are very important but they do not comprise the essence of spiritual care, which is often intangible with outcomes that are unknown, as will be very clear to anyone working in that area. The more meaningful aspects of spirituality and spiritual care, such as ways of being with people or empathy, are far harder to quantify or measure.

Although health care chaplaincy has produced standards for competent practice (NHS Training Directorate 1993) difficulties remain in linking these to actual practice, particularly as the concept of professional practice is at an early stage of development in chaplaincy services. The following examples do suggest that such organisational tools have the potential to promote spiritual care. Whipp (2001, pp.58–66) links audit to theological reflection and describes how an audit cycle can be used to improve patient care, including spiritual care. Kerry (2001, pp.118–32) describes a process that used such benchmarks to develop a local framework for competence that is encouraging as well as challenging for the staff involved. Although specifically developed for chaplains, the themes and approach could usefully be transferred to other professional groups involved in providing spiritual care.

The nature of spirituality makes these issues particularly apparent but in reality I hear similar arguments about other areas of health care. Working as a dietitian, I value the insights audit provides about our service yet audits never seem to reflect the whole of what we do. It is often the intangible, I would say spiritual, aspects of any health-related activity that are missing; the disquieting conversation about why to bother eating that leads to a change of heart; the moment of connection with a client that creates a new understanding or the motivation to change. As we have already discussed, measurable outcomes tend to skim the surface of spirituality, providing a useful minimum when the deeper reality usually offers so much more. That minimum is not unimportant but it is limited; recognised as a small contribution such results have value; taken to encompass the whole of holistic care they are distinctly lacking!

Outlining the difficulties of measuring outcomes in holistic care does not reduce the need for such care to be effective and well grounded, it simply asks questions about what exactly that means. In reality, the emphasis on wholeness and well-being should be seen as complementary to the emphasis on standards, guidelines and policies, reminding health care practitioners of the limitations of an isolated scientific approach. Spirituality cannot be reduced to just another task, just as improved spiritual care will not be achieved by another training package; something more is required. The opportunity for health care teams to learn together about spirituality might also lead them to discover new ways of researching that experience and all that arises from it.

8

Conclusion:
The Journey Continues

Returning to the idea of a journey, this book and the work to which it relates is the result of my own personal and professional journey within health care. These questions and ideas about spirituality grew as I worked within a palliative care team and I will always be glad that I was able to explore them more deeply in that context. Working in palliative care was a significant step in this journey, a change of direction that provided an enormous challenge to my thinking about spirituality. My whole understanding of spirituality needed to be re-examined and re-applied and that eventually led to fundamental changes in my own life as well as the way I worked. Talking to other members of the health care team was an important part of that process; conversations about spirituality often began rather diffidently but once we got beyond our initial uncertainty people expressed interest and enthusiasm about this subject. These conversations, formal and informal, encouraged me to think more deeply and widely than I could have done alone. Other people saw things differently, drew on different experiences and gently challenged ideas I would have taken for granted. Most of all, these travelling companions helped me stay in touch with reality and avoid getting lost or giving up when I seemed to be getting nowhere. My understanding of spirituality, indeed my whole approach to health care, has been profoundly affected by these experiences but the effects spread more widely than my own personal development. This journey of discovery took place in the context of a working health care team;

our shared exploration had a marked effect on that team as a whole as well as individual members of it. Later, through the development of a learning module about spirituality, our experiences began to affect staff and volunteers in the wider health care community.

This book has been an opportunity to share with a wider audience something of what we learnt. It has grown out of my concern that health care professionals should have a more grounded understanding of human spirituality, one that is an integral part of everyday practice as well as a nice theoretical idea. My experience of learning about spirituality was based in health care but it is clear that there is similar interest in other areas of work. Many of the themes discussed here could also be applied in other contexts – for example, in education. That learning process has been my main emphasis, rather than focusing primarily on the nature of spirituality. Understanding key issues such as holistic care, spirituality and spiritual care is important but much has been written about such issues already. I have been more interested to consider how we can learn about spirituality in a way that actually makes a difference to how health care teams work. My experience of learning about spirituality within just such a team has been used throughout the book with the intention of providing practical applications and illuminating theoretical ideas. This book is not a self-directed learning programme, although it can be used to develop the reader's understanding and ideas; nor is it an outline for a group learning programme, although again the ideas presented here could be used to help health care teams develop their own learning programmes. Rather it provides a practical outline of how learning about spirituality can occur within health care teams and the potential effect this can have on practice. This final chapter will provide an overview of the themes of the book.

Spirituality and the holistic approach

It is easy to speak superficially about holistic care, much harder to actually work in a holistic way. While the holistic approach is certainly not a new idea in health care, holism seems to be a way of working that has somehow been lost among the other issues that currently preoccupy modern health care. I suspect that most health care practitioners aim to work in a holistic way but the evidence we have suggests this theoretical ambition is rarely linked to actual practice. Human spirituality, in particular, is widely neglected in health care and this has a significant impact on the holistic approach. Perhaps that is not surprising given the context; the practical provision of holistic health care is beset with difficulties in the rapidly changing world in which we live and work. As we have explored earlier in this book, the failure to understand spirituality is not an isolated problem in health care but is linked to historical developments in the wider world. Human beings in the western world seem to have lost sight of the human spirit in their quest for a brave new world. Now, disillusioned by the limitations of science and technology but no longer willing to defer to authorities such as religion, people are once again interested in spirituality without knowing quite what that means. Health care is one of the areas where this uncertainty provides an uncomfortable context for a quite specific need for understanding and action.

At the heart of the holistic approach is such a seemingly simple idea; people are whole beings, each an inseparable amalgam of body, mind and spirit (or however those elements are labelled). Understanding and making space for the complexities of such human integration is never going to be easy but, it seems to me, the spiritual element is the area most easily misunderstood or neglected. Exploring and trying to understand this most intangible aspect of humanity may bring back into focus our overall perception of the holistic approach as well as increasing our understanding of spirituality itself. Our failure to understand and attend to spirituality is much more than just an interesting theoretical difficulty; it has a detrimental effect on health care practice and outcomes. This alone must surely encourage a renewal of interest in spirituality by health care professionals of all persuasions and a determination to uphold its integral place in holistic care. If the spiritual dimension really is central to every human being, then its effect on health and well-being cannot be ignored or forgotten. If we understand spirituality, for example, in terms of values, meaning or hope, these things inevitably influence health care in all but the most basic situations. A cut finger will probably heal without too much notice being taken of someone's spirituality, but dislocation of life caused by a long-term condition such as renal disease or by the sudden crisis of acute surgery soon make the links between spirituality and health more apparent. Jolted out of their normal life routines, people in such a situation may be unable to continue the work or hobbies that give life meaning. Foreseeing the strain this health crisis will place on relationships with family and friends, they may fear losing their connections with other people. Within all this, they are forced to realise that life, their own life, is more fragile than they had thought. All these, and many more, can be labelled as spiritual issues that health care professionals ignore at their peril.

Clients and health care professionals will make decisions and behave in ways that are affected by their beliefs and values, however much they are aware of that influence. Similarly the outcomes of health care, including the effectiveness of treatment, will also be affected by this essential part of our humanity, whether we recognise it or not. Health care teams need to be aware of the influence of spirituality on people's lives and learn how to recognise and take account of this in all aspects of their work. In order to do this, we must find ways of integrating the holistic approach into current health care practice. This means allowing for changes in health care such as increasing specialism and the growing emphasis on multi-professional team work, as well as changing health care concerns. Challenges such as patient choice and new technology, as well as changing disease patterns and ways of working, all contribute to the complexity of developing a truly holistic approach within health care. All these things present opportunities to develop an effective form of holistic and spiritual care as well as potential barriers to that happening. This book has explored spirituality as a specific element within holistic care, taking the view that spirituality is right at the heart of this process and not just an occasional addition. It is my belief that a better understanding of spirituality within health care is the key to a more widespread and practical rediscovery of the holistic approach.

Learning about spirituality in the multi-professional team

For historical and other reasons, spirituality is frequently connected to religion and this affects how both are regarded. Generally considered a very personal and private issue, spirituality is brought into a more public domain in the context of health care while still retaining some of the awkwardness attached to religion. Health care teams intending to work holistically need to overcome this awkwardness if they are to develop the shared understanding of spirituality that will allow them to explore spirituality with each other and with clients. Spirituality seems to integrate rather than divide by its very nature, straddling the artificial boundaries we erect between different aspects of our lives: between life and work, personal and private, patient and staff. Hence its importance as an integrating element for health care teams aiming to work holistically, but also the difficulty of practising in this way. Opportunities to learn about spirituality need to help health care staff traverse the additional boundary between theory and practice; there are plenty of interesting theoretical ideas about the nature of spirituality and spiritual care but unless some of this theory becomes embedded in practice nothing much will change and that would be a pity.

If spirituality is really such an integral element of health care, the whole health care team needs to be able to recognise and respond to spiritual needs. Despite much interest and discussion about spirituality in health care, the evidence we have suggests that health care teams do not tend to recognise or respond to spiritual need in practice. Even where individual health care professionals recognise a client's spiritual concerns, they often feel unable to respond directly. The most common response when spiritual concerns are expressed is to refer to a chaplain; a very relevant response for some clients but excluding for others and not always immediately available. How much better for the whole health care team to be aware of this element of their practice, able to recognise and respond to spiritual need in all clients and all situations. Sometimes this response would indeed mean referring on, perhaps to a chaplain or spiritual adviser, but at other times it would mean listening and staying with people as they struggle with those concerns for themselves. Where the whole team is involved in this way, a shared understanding of spirituality and spiritual care ensures a more considered and consistent approach to issues such as assessment and treatment, as well as overall approach. The process of developing and owning that shared understanding, as this book has discussed, can develop the confidence health care professionals need in order to become involved in spiritual care themselves. A shared understanding can also help the wider team recognise and value the broad and varied nature of spirituality and spiritual care. Spiritual care is not just about talking, or listening, but underpins many supportive aspects of health care. Health care teams need to reflect this breadth of involvement in spiritual care in the way they approach and organise opportunities to learn about spirituality.

Moving spirituality from a personal concern to a more public arena raises an inherent difficulty about the language we use. Spirituality is difficult to put into words; its meaning is complex and many layered, not easily reduced to neat formulae. This makes it harder to talk about but at the same time even more important to try; as we articulate our thoughts and experiences related to spirituality we learn more about what we think as well as what others think. Bringing discussions about spirituality out into the open in this way challenges ideas that are often taken for granted, and paves the way for greater clarity and a deeper understanding. This process can be difficult, even painful, as long-held or precious ideas are exposed to public view and dissected in order to gain greater understanding. This difficulty is intensified by the widespread reluctance to talk about spirituality and religion in public; this is changing as the idea of spirituality becomes more widely accepted but an understandable reluctance remains. Opportunities to explore spirituality need to occur in a supportive as well as a challenging environment. Too often discussions about spirituality become a polarised argument about religion or science, none of which helps develop the deeper understanding of spirituality needed in health care. The experience of the groups I worked with, as discussed in this book, suggests it is possible to overcome these difficulties and that this process will benefit the health care team. Given the right context, exploring spirituality with other people can lead to a greater confidence and awareness about spirituality, something that is personally and professionally enriching for the whole health care team.

Developing opportunities to talk about spirituality

A health care team that recognises the importance of the holistic approach, and accepts that this includes spirituality, is ready to start talking about what that means in actual practice. An opportunity for the health care team to explore spirituality together is an important step towards making the holistic approach a reality for that team. Establishing the necessary safe but challenging environment in which to learn about spirituality takes time and energy although I believe those resources will be well spent. Individuals who take part in this sort of exploration will, to some extent, be opening up their inner life to scrutiny and therefore making themselves vulnerable. Such a venture is not to be undertaken lightly or forced upon people but will need to be introduced cautiously. Careful thought also needs to be given to the format and facilitation of the group; done well this process will enliven and enrich those who take part, as well as benefitting the teams to which they belong; done badly, it could damage individuals and fracture the whole health care team.

The principles of adult and continuing education, particularly those of reflective practice, provide the essential foundations for this exploratory process. These may not be familiar to all health care practitioners, particularly those who trained some time ago, and it will be helpful for anyone undertaking an exploration of spirituality to revise some key principles before leaping into more specific content. Discussions about spirituality require the creation of a safe space, where each individual's beliefs and ideas are respected even where those views differ from other people's. With this acceptance of differing perspectives comes the recognition that it is valuable to listen to different viewpoints with an open mind and careful attention. That may not be easy given the complexity of spirituality and the inherent difficulties of talking about it. Time at the outset invested in exploring the aim of the group, agreeing the approach and ethos as well as setting practical ground rules will be of benefit later when discussions turn towards more personal and contentious topics. It takes time for trust to be established within a learning group, even within the context of a familiar team, particularly if the approach taken is different from the group's usual way of working. Learning about spirituality is not the same as learning about new clinical knowledge or techniques, partly because it affects people personally but also because of the nature of spirituality. In time, given that a safe space is established, individuals will become more able to speak openly about their beliefs and ideas – for example, by saying when they are not sure what something means, asking questions or admitting misunderstanding and uncertainty. As a secure context for learning becomes established, individuals will also be able to challenge each other in ways that are not confrontational. I have laboured the need for a safe but challenging environment in which to learn because exploring a topic like spirituality could cause irreparable damage if such preliminaries are not given due attention. Getting the environment (in its broadest sense) right is vital if real learning about spirituality is to take place and it may also help with learning in other areas.

The environment is affected by a number of things, including practical issues such as timing and physical space, facilitation and content. The principles of working with groups provide a helpful framework, so that it is clear from the start that even within an established team, the group will need to develop a level of trust that goes beyond that usually required as it settles into this new area of learning. A group will need adequate time, perhaps more than expected, to become established so that participants are comfortable enough with each other to speak about their own ideas and begin to challenge each other. Meeting regularly over a period of time also allows group members to apply those discussions to actual practice, bringing their reflections back to subsequent group meetings in order to refine and develop their thinking even further. Learning about spirituality is not something to be rushed, whatever pressure there may be to do so. A new insight or idea may arrive in seconds but that insight often stems from the much slower process of reflection as participants listen and ponder, hearing each other's stories and their own in a new way, perhaps struggling to understand what someone means; all that simply takes time.

Previous experience of learning, roles within the team and other similar issues all affect the way in which this process occurs. Tuckman's recognition that groups go through the stages of forming, storming and norming before they start performing is worth remembering if groups meeting to explore spirituality are going to thrive and develop. It is also worth considering the expected life span of the group at the beginning rather than allow it to either continue indefinitely or gradually fizzle out. The facilitator's role remains the key to such details; teams will need to think carefully about who takes on this role and the support the facilitator will need from the rest of the group. When health care teams learn together, those involved will be adults who bring a wealth of experience as a resource for their learning. This is no less so when learning about spirituality but it is important to recognise that prior experience may be positive or negative. Adults may also be more fixed in their ideas and, therefore, less open to exploration and debate, the very attributes that are particularly helpful when exploring spirituality. Widely divergent views about spirituality are likely to occur when learning involves the wider health care team rather than just interested individuals. This is one of the strengths of such a group as it provides a wide scope of experience but it also provides a potential source of conflict. The learning group, with the help of the facilitator, will need to respond to such differences and ensure they are used to the benefit of learning rather than becoming a source of disruption or dispute. The key to that is for the group to agree and then adhere to ground rules that respect and value different ideas; it is the difficult task of the facilitator to ensure they do so.

The reflective and experiential approach to learning, such as I have advocated, aims to work with the learner's own experience as well as theoretical concepts. Experienced health care professionals may see clearly the relevance of spirituality to their life and work, another characteristic of adult learners, but they may also expect that learning will give them answers to the problems they experience. All my discussions have indicated that a problem-solving approach is not really the place to start when learning about spirituality; rather the aim is to integrate theory with practice in a way that deepens understanding and confidence. Sometimes that will help clients resolve their difficulties but, perhaps more commonly, it will help people recognise that there are some problems that cannot be solved. Helping health care professionals accept their limitations without disengaging from clients is also a valid piece of learning. This may be part of the equalising effect of spirituality, a recognition that we are all human and that learning is a two-way process where the health care professional can learn from the client, as well as the other way round. Grounding learning about spirituality in experience, including difficult experience, as well as relating it to theoretical concepts not only strengthens the link with practice but also raises motivation and interest. This is learning that can make a real difference to human life and not something limited to ivory-towered academia.

Schon's image of learning in the 'swampy lowlands where messy confusing problems defy technical solution' (1988, p.3) has become familiar within discussions about reflective practice. This is a powerful image that resonates with many working in health care where the really important problems we face often do seem messy and confusing. Reflective practice aims to integrate theory and practice in the actual workplace, where feelings and attitudes are irrevocably intertwined with theoretical ideas and techniques. Spirituality, although far from being simply a problem to be solved, has that same sense of being hard to define. I hope I have demonstrated that spirituality is concerned with real issues about what it is to be human for both client and carer; issues that go to the very heart of health care practice. Reflecting together on these deeper issues, as individuals and as a whole group, health care teams can develop new insights to create a more substantial web of understanding. I do not think this will ever mean that spirituality is neatly defined and pinned down but it may help those who explore it in this way to be more comfortable with their lack of answers. Groups may find it helpful, if challenging, to use different learning opportunities as a stimulus for discussions; thinking, for example, about images from film or theatre can bring a new dimension to ideas about spirituality. Being open to different ways of learning will help the group to be open to new ideas, recognising that there is more here than they know or understand, in itself a valuable piece of learning about spirituality.

Continuing professional development is essential in health care as in other areas of professional practice. In a rapidly changing world it is vital to continue learning about all aspects of health care practice. Much continuing professional development in health care focuses on new clinical knowledge or techniques, but increased self-awareness and understanding of personal attitudes can also be part of learning. I have been concerned to emphasise that continuing professional development also applies to somewhat nebulous ideas about holistic care and spirituality. These ideas relate directly to the art of health care, intended to work hand in hand with scientific knowledge and practical technique. Without an understanding of spirituality, for example, new technical knowledge about an enteral feed or medication will be so much more limited. To learn about a new treatment within the context of understanding the client as a whole is a richer and more beneficial development than simply learning a new technique in isolation. A wide variety of factors influence how new techniques are received by clients; spirituality, if we describe it in terms of meaning and purpose, hope or connections with others, will affect client motivation as well as their acceptance of new ideas. Health care professionals who recognise this deeper level in their practice will be able to see new developments in a substantial context, as if in colours rather than greyscale. An understanding of spirituality and holistic care should be an integral part of all learning in health care but it also, at least for the moment, requires more focused attention in its own right to reduce the effect of recent neglect and confusion. The exploration of spirituality and spiritual care that I have been advocating is not intended to be isolated from other aspects of holistic care but is rather a necessary preparation for working holistically.

Understanding spirituality

Health care teams wishing to work more holistically and to integrate spirituality into their practice need to prepare by spending time attending to spirituality themselves. The growing and wide-ranging interest in spirituality in the wider world makes this focused attention imperative in order to find some agreement and clarity about this subject. Within the existing confusion, it is helpful to identify repeating themes about the nature of spirituality; these offer openings to be explored by health care teams. In earlier chapters I have considered a number of recurring themes about spirituality that emerge from the literature as well as the experience of groups that I worked with. The experience of those groups was that it was possible to find some agreement about key issues even among our wide-ranging ideas about spirituality. Even where individuals expressed their own spirituality in very different ways, it was still helpful, and possible, to identify key shared ideas. Although this process was difficult, and at times uncomfortable, it eventually helped us develop a stronger, shared understanding about spirituality that began to affect our practice as individuals and as a team.

An initial area of agreement is the perception of spirituality as a unique, innate potential within each individual. Hardly a radical idea, it was only as we began to explore the application of this in health care practice that its significance really began to appear. Spirituality that is an integral element of each and every person should be considered within everyone. An innate spirituality also becomes something each person will attend to at different stages in their life; relevant to health care professionals as well as clients, to the many and not the select few. This founding principle begins to explain why spirituality is so pervasive in our thinking about health care; relevant to health promotion, active treatment of disease and palliative care, to staff as well as clients and carers, and across all age groups from birth to death; it affects the physical environment as well as subtle questions of attitude and approach. Health care, like education, provides a moment when individuals are more open to learn about spirituality. Where this exploration of spirituality has been neglected in the past, illness may remind people, perhaps for the first time or in new ways, that they are spiritual beings. This experience stimulates questions as people pause and reflect on their experience, spiritual questions about who they are and what they are doing. This may lead to helpful coping strategies but it can also provoke a spiritual crisis that simply adds to the confusion of physical or mental distress. It is important for members of the health care team to be aware of this process in clients as well as in themselves and their colleagues, so they can provide support where required as well as notice the effect on health and well-being. Developing this sort of awareness is an essential part of learning in its widest sense, vital for continuing professional development but also for personal development.

Spirituality can be understood as the essence of what it is to be human, an integrating force that leads people to look inward to understand better who they are but also to look outward to other people and beyond that to transcendent values and beliefs. If spirituality is related to the human search for meaning and purpose, to work out what really matters, it becomes part of our continuing attempt to make sense of life, to find hope and a connection with others and the wider world. My spirit becomes woven through everything that I do and am, from everyday tasks and activities to bigger issues of identity and relationship. My work, my home, my health, my choices in life, my relationships, my ideas and thoughts, can all be related to my spirit in ways that continue to emphasise my wholeness. It is important to understand that people may express their spirituality in many different ways over time rather than fitting one preferred or more acceptable pattern. We should expect to see the human spirit grow and develop, much as we would expect to see human bodies and minds develop.

Health care staff who wish to work holistically will benefit personally and professionally as they develop a robust understanding of spirituality through discussion with other members of the health care team. Having a basic shared understanding of spirituality that can be expressed with a degree of comfort and personal understanding supports the integration of spirituality into everyday practice and is a necessary foundation for the provision of spiritual care. A healthy spirit is an essential part of human well-being, saving people from anomie and distress and contributing significantly to total health and well-being. Staff who elect to explore this area of health care may find themselves more aware of their own needs for a balanced life that includes opportunities to care for the spirit. This recognition of shared humanity and mutual need is one reason why spirituality is something of an equaliser in health care, an area where no one has all the answers and few would see themselves as an expert. These positive aspects of spirituality and spiritual care need to be recognised as a force for good throughout health care, part of a holistic approach that benefits patients and staff alike.

Spiritual care

Having a more confident and discerning understanding of spirituality has benefits in many areas, such as health promotion and staff support as well as beyond health care, but there remains a more specific need for spiritual care and support in illness. Spiritual care, as outlined in this book, is about providing a safe and hospitable place where it is possible to explore human spirituality within the context of holistic care. Far from always being a problem, spirituality is simply an integral and integrating element within each person, a potential source of distress but also of strength and well-being that should not be ignored by those involved in health care. Health care staff who are comfortable with this area of their work, including their own personal spirituality, will be able to recognise and respond appropriately when clients raise issues or concerns that can be linked to spirituality. They can also be proactive about considering spirituality as part of overall care. Opportunities to explore spirituality together, as outlined in this book, enable the development of a shared understanding and approach within health care teams as well as giving individuals a rare opportunity to explore their own spirituality in relation to their work. Again, this will take time and energy but, if the outcome is a truly holistic integrated approach that is better for clients and staff, then that time will surely be well spent.

Something of this shared approach needs to extend across the wider health care team rather than be limited to selected groups of staff. Some of the most practically involved members of the health care team, as described in Box 2.1 (p.24), lift a client's spirits by being themselves in a way that is not easily labelled. Being human is effectively at the heart of spiritual care, operating through therapeutic relationships as well as more practical forms of support. Yet, essential as this is, health care staff may find their humanity battered and bruised by the very experience of working in health care settings. Protective boundaries intended to help health care staff and clients alike can become impenetrable and practical tasks overwhelming, so that there is little opportunity to remember these more intangible aspects of health care. My experience has been that spending time reflecting on spirituality with colleagues made it easier to recognise and value the part I myself play in my health care practice. Sharing that human vulnerability with other members of the health care team opens up the possibilities of receiving as well as giving support and acceptance. In reality it is impossible not to bring our humanity into our health care practice; increased self-awareness can make that a positive experience for clients and health care staff alike.

The provision of spiritual care requires a context where spirituality is simply an integral element of the whole health care service. An understanding of spirituality should affect decisions about a wide range of issues at both a strategic and operational level, including staff, activity and surroundings. Spiritual care becomes something in which all the team are involved and for which they need to be equipped. If spirituality is essentially about being human, spiritual care is more about who we are than what we do, about offering our shared humanity to others rather than any particular role or activity. Understanding ourselves and other people better, with particular reference to understanding spirituality, is the best preparation for providing spiritual care and this requires continuing learning. Where spirituality is an integral part of the whole of health care provision this will be demonstrated in myriad large and small ways to reflect that underlying ethos. More practical aspects of spiritual care may include a wide range of services such as listening, divertional or creative therapies and meeting religious needs. These activities can never comprise the whole of spiritual care and need to be provided in the understanding that spiritual care is more about who we are than what we do. It is quite different, and likely to be rather hollow, simply to provide certain activities in the hope that these will be an opportunity for spiritual care; providing spiritual care may simply be about acknowledging and valuing spirituality in all that we do.

Assessment of spirituality should be a core part of spiritual care, ensuring a proactive, consistent approach across the health care team. Yet in reality it is not easy to carry out any set form of assessment; spirituality seems too personal to raise in this formal way, not least because the language used is so complex and easily misunderstood. Reflective learning to develop a shared understanding of spirituality enables health care staff to recognise and respond to clients' spirituality in more diffuse but no less proactive ways. Again, health care staff who are comfortable with the concepts of spirituality and alert to their own spiritual nurture are more likely to be able to work in this way. This also ensures that assessment is integrated with other forms of support, and underpinned by shared understanding and a collective approach.

Greater awareness of common themes within spirituality can lead to a more proactive approach to spiritual care – for example, discussions about what gives life meaning, connections with others or religious practices can be included in routine assessment. Sources of meaning and purpose vary widely between individuals but lack of meaning is usually viewed as a sign of poor health. The ways in which illness so often threatens our sense of meaning and purpose, as well as our relationships, contributes significantly to the distress people experience when they or members of their family become ill. Other key themes that can be used in this way include hope, connection with others, and beliefs and values. While religion is now recognised as only one expression of spirituality it remains an important one for many people. As well as ensuring a framework within which to develop and nurture the human spirit, religion provides a link with a well-established community of shared values and beliefs, although these will be expressed differently in specific faith communities.

Talking about spirituality is important for health care staff who wish to provide spiritual care; similarly, listening when clients decide to talk openly about spirituality can be important in spiritual care. This does not mean expecting to have deep spiritual conversations with every client or colleague, rather it is about remembering spirituality in all that we do. Of course, spiritual growth does not occur simply by talking about it, indeed silence may be more fruitful. However, the opportunity to reflect out loud, even if that is difficult, is likely to be an important part of unpacking other opportunities, helping to acknowledge what is going on and learn from it. Reflecting on meaning or purpose, hope, connection with others, can all be seen as part of exploring spirituality and therefore supporting spiritual care. To return to the metaphor of the journey that has been a regular theme, spiritual care is about offering to share part of clients' journeys. Offering them a lift towards my destination or suggesting they try a different mode of transport could easily waste their time and energy; we cannot do the travelling for them. We cannot even necessarily be a guide for the way; rather we are companions on the road who may provide support for a time. Even to do that, we must be travelling ourselves and we will all gain as we listen to each other's stories along the way.

Conclusion

This journey, affecting me personally as well as professionally, comes to a new divergence of ways with the completion of this book. I still work in the health service, although no longer in palliative care, and am still involved in an Anglican church. Working now in more acute health care I still see the benefits of exploring spirituality within health care teams, benefits for the team itself as well as for clients. Working holistically, with spirituality as an integral part of such an approach, is not the easiest way to work, but it remains for me the very essence of health care.

Appendix 1:
A Short Course on Spirituality

The short course on spirituality referred to in this book was first run as part of the Manchester Palliative Care Education (MPaCE) initiative. This programme of skills-based short courses was developed by a consortium of palliative care providers in south Manchester. Modules covered a wide range of topics and were specifically designed to enable practitioners to develop skills relevant to palliative care. MPaCE courses, including the spirituality course, are still being provided and more details can be obtained from:

The Institute for Learning and Development
St Ann's Hospice
St Ann's Road North
Heald Green
Cheadle
Cheshire SK8 3SZ
Tel: 0161 489 3615

Appendix 2: Suggested Outline for Groups Wishing to Explore Spirituality

Introductory session

It is helpful to offer an initial open introductory session to which the whole health care team is invited. This gives potential participants an opportunity to explore the idea of the group before making a definite commitment to be involved. This session should focus on exploring the aim of the group, ground rules, membership, approach and the role of the facilitator. An icebreaker (see the example below) may be useful even if the group is part of an established team. An introductory activity – for example, brainstorming ideas about what spirituality is and is not – could be used to give people an idea of what to expect. By the end of this session people should feel confident that the group will provide a safe space in which to explore spirituality and understand the reflective and exploratory approach that will be used. The aim and ground rules should be reviewed at the first formal session of the group.

Icebreaker: Each person asks the question 'Where have you come from?' of another person in the group, who should respond by saying something about the physical, mental or spiritual journey that has brought him or her to this moment. Move round until most people have spoken to each other *but* they must talk about a different aspect of this journey each time.

Plan for individual sessions

Opening: Each session should begin with a period of open reflection where participants can raise relevant incidents, items for the bulletin board or other contributions. This may feel uncomfortable initially but helps establish an open, reflective approach.

Main focus: A series of key themes can be introduced using some of the examples below. Initially themes would be introduced by the tutors with some background material or an activity to start the discussion but later other participants should also be involved. There should be an emphasis on linking theory and practice, encouraging people to look at theoretical material, such as relevant journal articles, but also drawing on their personal experience.

Closing: It may help to end sessions with an agreed activity, such as a few minutes' quiet or a guided reflection, or simply time for participants to write in their journals.

Suggested activities

Spirituality and the holistic approach: Can orthodox health care really be holistic? In what ways might spirituality provide a key to a more holistic approach? Reflect together on this quotation:

> We generally feel somewhat embarrassed to mention things like love, joy, peace, sense of purpose, connectedness, reverence for living or achieving one's full potential in the context of health promotion programs. Should we not strive to broaden our concept of health promotion to include these kinds of issues? After all what is life worth if there is no love in it? Or joy? Are we only interested in prolonging life and unclogging arteries? (Chapman 1986, p.38)

Spirituality and the multi-professional team: What are the benefits and difficulties of exploring spirituality within health care teams? List the roles that are included in the multi-professional health care team; how might each person be involved in spirituality? Discuss your response to the reflection in Box 2.1 (p.39) and any implications for the health care team.

Defining spirituality: Look at some definitions of spirituality (for example, those given in Box 5.1, p.85). Ask the group to discuss how they feel about each of the definitions and how they fit with the experience of people in the group. Group members should reflect on how ideas about spirituality seem to have changed during their working life and what has led to those changes. Consider what difference it would make to day-to-day health care if spirituality were fully accepted as an innate potential in every person as suggested in Chapter 5. What implications does this view have for group members' personal and professional lives?

Understanding spirituality: There are many articles and papers on the nature of spirituality, some of which are referred to in this book. Choose a selection of articles looking at key themes such as those outlined in Chapter 5. Each member of the group (or working in pairs) should read and reflect on the ideas within one particular article, critically appraising the content and using that to generate discussion by the whole group. This activity may take several weeks as differing themes are explored. Some groups may also wish to explore the research basis for spirituality, but beware of becoming too theoretical and losing the link with practical experience.

Talking about spirituality: Each participant should prepare for the session by reflecting on any discussion about spirituality within the health care team where he or she is based. It may help to keep a rough diary for a few weeks recording any relevant issues related to spirituality, such as conversations with clients or staff.

- What discussions occur within the team that seem to relate to spirituality?
- Are these formal or informal?
- Where do they happen and who is involved?
- How would a shared understanding of spirituality affect these discussions?

Picturing spirituality: It is sometimes easier to use metaphorical (picture) language to talk about spirituality; for example, images such as the journey or a garden. Everyone in the group should think of an image that reflects their ideas about spirituality. Talk about these images together, noticing any similarities or differences. Can you think of other metaphors used by clients or health care staff in this way and what might these images be trying to say? Reflect on why metaphorical language, stories, pictures or poems might help people talk about spirituality and related issues such as death.

Telling tales: Encourage participants to reflect on their own individual spiritual resources and prepare to talk to the group about some aspect of their own spiritual story. This should be something they are comfortable discussing with other people and can arise from any aspect of their own experience. They may wish to bring a visual aid, piece of music or other artefact to help them tell the story and can use any style they wish to tell the story. This activity may be used in the final session of the group or may be spread over several sessions as an ending activity.

Spiritual care in practice: To prepare for the session, each member of the group should select an incident with a client that raises questions about spirituality, and reflect on the following questions:

- What questions did it raise and why? Why are these spiritual questions?
- How did you respond to this incident?
- Did your professional training equip you for this experience?
- Did you discuss the incident with other team members and, if so, in what context?
- In what ways did this experience affect you personally and professionally?

This could be used in the initial part of the session for a number of weeks with participants taking turns to share their reflections on a particular incident with the whole group. This leads into discussion by the whole group looking for common themes and aiming to learn from each other's experiences.

Recognising spirituality: Brainstorm all the ways in which spirituality could be an integral part of health care provision; for example, environment, buildings, care planning, assessments, treatments, resources, staffing. Participants should then review how many of these options are currently an integral part of the health care settings where they work. What more could be done or what could be done better? Look for practical suggestions to try to plan how they could be included.

Spiritual assessment: Look at the strengths, weaknesses, opportunities and threats (SWOT) of using a spiritual assessment tool in health care. If possible, review a number of actual assessment tools, including any that participants are using, or discuss some of the questions included in Box 6.1 (p.121) and how these could be used in practice. Individual participants may like to try using some of these questions with each other and discuss how it felt both to ask and answer each question.

Back to my health care team: Reflect on how spirituality is integrated into the health care provided by your team, describing the practical ways it affects the team's activity. It may be helpful to consider whether spiritual aspects of care are discussed openly by team members with each other and with clients or carers, and how spiritual care is offered. What makes it difficult or easy to discuss spirituality within this particular team? It would be interesting to explore how participants' experiences differ within the same team or different teams.

The above suggestions are only the beginning. You are sure to have ideas of your own.

References

Adam, D. (2005) 'Meditation leads to longer life.' *Education Guardian,* 2 May.

Amenta, M. (1997) 'Spiritual care: the heart of palliative nursing.' *International Journal of Palliative Nursing 3,* 1, 4.

Bandolier (1997) 'Old Curiosity Shop: the power of prayer.' 46, 6, 1–3. www.jr2.ox.ac.uk/bandolier.band46.b46-6.html

Benson, H. with Stark, M. (1996) *Timeless Healing.* London: Simon & Schuster.

Berger, P. (1969) *The Social Reality of Religion.* London: Faber & Faber (also published in 1967 as *The Sacred Canopy*).

Billington, M. (1999) 'Barnstormers.' *Guardian, Saturday Review,* 11 December, 4.

Bradshaw, A. (1994) *Lighting The Lamp: The Spiritual Dimension of Nursing Care.* Royal College of Nursing Research Series, Middlesex: SCUTARI Press.

Burnard, P. (1990) 'Learning to care for the spirit.' *Nursing Standard 4,* 18, 38–39.

Burne, J. (2000) 'Healing in harmony.' *Guardian Weekend,* 26 February, 9–17.

Burne, J. (2004) 'Sick? But I'm just not the type.' *Independent Review,* 14 June, 10–11.

Burton, L.N. (1998) 'The spiritual dimension of palliative care.' *Seminars in Oncology Nursing 14,* 2, 121–128.

Candy, P.C. (1986) 'The eye of the beholder: metaphor in adult education research.' *International Journal of Life Long Education 5,* 2, 89–111.

Canter, P.H. and Ernst, E. (2004) 'Insufficient evidence to conclude whether or not transcendental meditation decreases blood pressure: results of a systematic review of randomised control trials.' *Journal of Hypertension 22,* 11, 2049–54.

Catterall, R.A., Cox, M., Greet, B., Sankey, J. and Griffiths, G. (1998) 'The assessment and audit of spiritual care.' *International Journal of Palliative Nursing 4,* 4, 162–168.

Chapman, L. (1986) 'Spiritual health: a component missing from health promotion.' *American Journal of Health Promotion,* Summer, 38–41.

Church Times (2005) 'Petals fall to recollect tsunami victims.' 13 May, 3.

Cobb, M. and Robshaw, V. (eds) (1998) *The Spiritual Challenge of Health Care.* London: Churchill Livingstone.

Cornette, K. (1997) 'For whenever I am weak, I am strong.' *International Journal of Palliative Nursing 3,* 1, 6–13.

Davie, G. and Cobb, M. (1998) 'Faith and belief: a sociological perspective.' In M. Cobb and V. Robshaw (eds) *The Spiritual Challenge of Health Care.* London: Churchill Livingstone.

De Henezal, M. (1997) (trans. C.B. Janeway) *Intimate Death.* London: Little, Brown & Company.

Department of Health (1991) *The Patient's Charter.* London: HMSO.

Department of Health (1998) *A First Class Service: Quality in the new NHS.* London: HMSO.

Department of Health (2003a) *NHS Chaplaincy: Meeting the Religious and Spiritual Needs of Patients and Staff.* London: The Stationery Office.

Department of Health (2003b) *Building on the Best: Choice, Responsiveness and Equity in the NHS.* London: The Stationery Office.

Department of Health (2004a) *The NHS Improvement Plan: Putting People at the Heart of Public Services.* London: The Stationery Office.

Department of Health (2004b) *The Knowledge and Skills Framework.* London: The Stationery Office.

Don, M. (2001) 'Fighting shy.' *Observer Magazine,* 30 September, p.74.

Engquist, D.E., Short-DeGraff, M., Gliner, J. and Oltjenbruns, K. (1997) 'Occupational therapists' beliefs and practices with regard to spirituality.' *American Journal of Occupational Therapy 51,* 3, 173–180.

Frankl, V. (1964) (trans. Ilse Lasch) *Man's Search for Meaning.* London: Hodder & Stoughton.

Fredette, S.L. (1995) 'Breast cancer survivors: concerns and coping.' *Cancer Nursing 18,* 1, 35–46.

Georgesen, J. and Dungan, J.M. (1996) 'Managing spiritual distress in patients with advanced cancer pain.' *Cancer Nursing 19,* 5, 376–383.

Giske, T. (1995) 'Spiritual care in nursing practice.' *Christian Nurse International 11,* 4, 4–8.

Hall, B.A. (1997) 'Spirituality in terminal illness: an alternative view of theory.' *Journal of Holistic Nursing 15,* 1, 82–96.

Hall, J. (2000) 'Spiritual midwifery care: old practice for a new millennium.' *British Journal of Midwifery 8,* 2, 82.

Hardy, A. (1979) *The Spiritual Nature of Man.* Oxford: The Religious Experience Research Unit.

Harrison, J. and Burnard, P. (1993) 'Spirituality and nursing practice.' Aldershott: Avebury Press.

Hay, D. (1982) *Exploring Inner Space.* Middlesex: Penguin.

Hay, D. (1990) *Religious Experience Today.* London: Mowbray.

Heald, G. (2000) *Soul of Britain.* London: The Opinion Research Business.

Health Education Authority (1999) *Promoting Mental Health: The Role of Faith Communities – Jewish and Christian Perspectives.* London: Health Education Authority.

Healthcare Commission (2004) *State of Healthcare Report.* London: Healthcare Commission.

Heelas, P. and Woodhead, L. (2005) *The Spiritual Revolution: Why Religion is Giving Way to Spirituality.* Oxford: Blackwell Publishing.

Heron, J. (1996) *Co-operative Inquiry.* London: Sage.

Highfield, M.F. (1992) 'Spiritual health of oncology patients.' *Cancer Nursing 15,* 1, 1–8.

Highfield, M.F. (1997) 'Spiritual assessment across the cancer trajectory: methods and reflections.' *Seminars in Oncology Nursing 13*, 4, 237–241.

Highfield, M.F. and Cason, C. (1983) 'The spiritual needs of patients: are they recognised?' *Cancer Nursing 6*, 3, 187–192.

Hodge, D. (2005) 'Spiritual lifemaps: a client centred pictorial instrument for spiritual assessment, planning and intervention.' *Social Work 50*, 1, 77–88.

Holly, M.L. (1989) 'Reflective writing and the spirit of inquiry.' *Cambridge Journal of Education 19*, 1, 71–80.

Illich, I. (1976) *Limits to Medicine.* London: Marian Boyars Publishers Ltd.

Illman, J. (1998) 'You really can die of a broken heart but psalms and sermons could save you.' *Observer*, 17 May, 12.

Jenkins, D. (1997) Unpublished welcome address delivered at the Spirituality and Health conference, 30 September–2 October, Durham (from my notes).

Karpiak, I.E. (1992) 'Beyond competence: continuing education and the evolving self.' *The Social Worker 60*, 1, 53–57.

Kearney, M. (1996) *Mortally Wounded.* Dublin: Marino Books.

Keighley, T. (1997) 'Organisational structures and personal spiritual beliefs.' *International Journal of Palliative Nursing 3*, 1, 47–51.

Kelly, L. (1988) 'The ethics of caring: has it been discarded?' *Nursing Outlook 36*, 17.

Kerry, M. (2001) 'Towards competence: a narrative and framework for spiritual care givers.' In H. Orchard (ed.) *Spirituality in Health Care Contexts.* London: Jessica Kingsley Publishers.

King's College London (University of London) (2004) *Improving Supportive and Palliative Care for Adults with Cancer: Research Evidence.* Available at www.nice.org.uk

Labun, E. (1988) 'Spiritual care: an element in nursing care planning.' *Journal of Advanced Nursing 13*, 314–320.

Lash, J. (1998) *On Pilgrimage.* London: Bloomsbury Publishing Ltd.

Leedham, K. and Platt, K. (1998) 'Community cancer support: the Neil Cliffe Cancer Care Charity approach to supportive care.' *International Journal of Palliative Nursing 4*, 2, 58–64.

Levin, J.S., Larson, D.B. and Puchalski, C.M. (1997) 'Religion and spirituality in medicine: research and education.' *Journal of the American Medical Association 278*, 9, 792–793.

Little, W., Fowler, H.W. and Coulson, J. (1973) *The Shorter Oxford English Dictionary.* Oxford: Clarendon Press (with revisions by C.T. Onions and G.W.S Friedrichson).

Maddocks, M. (1988) *Twenty Questions about Healing.* London: SPCK.

McSherry, E. (1983) 'The scientific basis of whole person medicine.' *Journal of the American Scientific Affiliation*, December, 217–224.

McSherry, W. (1997) *A Descriptive Survey of Nurses' Perceptions of Spirituality and Spiritual Care* (unpublished MPhil thesis). Hull: University of Hull.

McSherry, W. (2000) *Spirituality in Nursing Practice: An Interactive Approach.* Edinburgh: Churchill Livingstone.

Mearns, D. and Thorne, B. (1999) *Person Centred Counselling In Action.* London: Sage Publications.

MHA Care Group (2005) MHA research on spirituality, at www.mha.org.uk

Murray, R.B. and Zentner, J.P. (1988) *Nursing Concepts for Health Promotion.* Hemel Hempstead: Prentice-Hall.

Narayanasamy, A. (1991) *Spiritual Care: A Resource Guide.* Lancaster: BKT Information Services Quay Publishing.

Narayanasamy, A. (1993) 'Nurses' awareness and educational preparation in meeting their patients' spiritual needs.' *Nurse Education Today 13,* 196–201.

Narayanasamy, A. (2004) 'The puzzle of spirituality for nursing: a guide to practical assessment.' *British Journal of Nursing 13,* 19, 28 October–10 November, 1140–1144.

National Association of Health Authorities and Trusts (1996) *Spiritual Care in the NHS.* Birmingham: NAHAT.

National Institute for Clinical Excellence (NICE) (2002) *Improving Outcomes in Breast Cancer* (manual update). Available at www.nice.org.uk

National Institute for Clinical Excellence (NICE) (2004) *Improving Supportive and Palliative Care for Adults with Cancer: Guidelines.* Available at www.nice.org.uk

Neuberger, J. (1999) 'Going beyond Medicine.' *NHS Magazine,* Summer, 22–23.

NHS Executive Northern and Yorkshire Chaplains and Pastoral Care Committee (1995) *Framework for Spiritual, Faith and Related Pastoral Care.* Leeds: Institute of Nursing, University of Leeds.

NHS Training Directorate (1993) *Health Care Chaplaincy Standards.* Bristol: NHS Training Directorate.

Oldnall, A. (1996) A Critical Analysis of Nursing: Meeting the Spiritual Needs of Patients. *Journal of Advanced Nursing 23,* pp.138–144.

Orchard, H. (2000) *Hospital Chaplaincy: Modern, Dependable?* (Research Reports 1). Sheffield: Lincoln Theological Research Institute.

Pattison, S. (2001) 'Dumbing down the spirit.' In H. Orchard (ed.) *Spirituality in Health Care Contexts.* London: Jessica Kingsley Publishers.

Post, S.G., Puchalski, C.M. and Larson, D.B. (2000) 'Physicians and patient spirituality: professional boundaries, competency and ethics.' *Annals of Internal Medicine 132,* 7, 578–583.

Post-White, J., Ceronsky, C., Kreitzer, M.J., Nickelson, K., Drew, D., Mackey, K.W., Koopmeiners, L. and Gutknecht, S. (1996) 'Hope, spirituality, sense of coherence and quality of life in patients with cancer', *Oncology Nursing Forum 23,* 10, 1571–1579.

Reason, P. and Heron, J. (1985) *Whole Person Medicine: A Co-operative Inquiry.* London: British Post Graduate Medical Federation and Human Potential Research Project.

Reason, P. and Rowan, J. (1981) *Human Inquiry: A Source Book of New Paradigm Research.* Chichester: John Wiley & Sons.

Redfern, A. (1999) *Ministry and Priesthood.* London: DLT.

Reed, P. (1987) 'Spirituality and well being in terminally ill hospitalised adults', *Research in Nursing and Health 10*, 335–344.

Renetzky, L. (1979) 'The fourth dimension: applications to the social services.' In D. Moberg (ed.) *Spiritual Well Being: Sociological Perspectives.* Washington: University Press of America.

Ross, L. (1994) 'Spiritual aspects of nursing.' *Journal of Advanced Nursing 19*, 439–447.

Ross, L. (1997a) 'The nurse's role in assessing and responding to patients' spiritual needs.' *International Journal of Palliative Nursing 3*, 1, 37–42.

Ross, L. (1997b) 'Elderly patients' perceptions of their spiritual needs and care: a pilot study.' *Journal of Advanced Nursing 26*, 710–715.

Ross, L. (1998) 'The nurse's role in spiritual care.' In M. Cobb and V. Robshaw (eds) *The Spiritual Challenge of Health Care.* London: Churchill Livingstone.

Royal College of Nursing Resource Guide (1998) *The Nursing Care of Older People from Black and Minority Ethnic Groups.* London: RCN.

Schon, D. (1988) *Educating the Reflective Practitioner: Towards a New Design for Teaching and Learning in the Professions.* London: Jossey Bass Publishers.

School of Health and Related Research (University of Sheffield) (2004) *Improving Supportive and Palliative Care for Adults with Cancer: Economic Review.* Available at www.nice.org.uk

Simsen, B. (1985) *Spiritual Needs and Resources in Illness and Hospitalisation* (unpublished MSc Thesis). Manchester: University of Manchester.

Simsen, B. (1986) 'The spiritual dimension.' *Nursing Times*, 26 November, 41–42.

Sloan, R.P., Bagiella, E. and Powell, T. (1999) 'Religion, spirituality and medicine.' *The Lancet 353*, 9153, 664–667.

Sloan, R.P., Bagiella, E., VandeCreek, L., Hover, M., Casalone, C., Hirsch, T.J., Hasan, Y., Kreger, R. and Poulos, P. (2000) 'Should physicians prescribe religious activities?' *The New England Journal of Medicine 342*, 25, 1913–1916.

Smith, M.E. (1999) 'Spiritual issues.' In J. Lugton and M. Kindlen (eds) *Palliative Care: The Nursing Role.* Edinburgh: Churchill Livingstone.

Somalai, A.M. and Heckman, T.G. (2000) 'Correlates of spirituality and well being in a community sample of people living with HIV disease.' *Mental Health, Religion and Culture 3*, 1, 57–70.

Speck, P., Higginson, I. and Addington-Hall, J. (2004) 'Spiritual needs in health care.' *British Medical Journal 329*, 123–124.

Spiritual Care Work Group of the International Work Group on Death, Dying and Bereavement (1990) 'Assumptions and principles of spiritual care.' *Death Studies 14*, 75–81.

Stoll, R. (1979) 'Guidelines for spiritual assessment.' *American Journal of Nursing 4*, 1574–1577.

Stoter, D. (1995) *Spiritual Aspects of Health Care.* London: Mosby.

Swinton, J. (2001) *Spirituality and Mental Health Care: Rediscovering a Forgotten Dimension.* London: Jessica Kingsley Publishers.

Taylor, E.J., Highfield, M. and Amenta, M. (1994) 'Attitudes and beliefs regarding spiritual care.' *Cancer Nursing 17*, 6, 479–487.

Tomalin, C. (2003) *Samuel Pepys: The Unequalled Self.* London: Penguin Books.

Townsend, P., Davidson, N. and Whitehead, M. (1990) *Inequalities in Health.* London: Penguin Books.

Tuckman, B. (1965) 'Development sequence in small groups.' *Psychological Bulletin LXIII*, 6.

Twycross, R.G. and Lack, S.A. (1990) *Therapeutics in Terminal Cancer.* Edinburgh: Churchill Livingstone.

Usher, R. (1993) 'Experiential learning or learning from experience, does it make a difference?' In D. Boud, R. Cohen and D. Walker (eds) *Using Experience for Learning.* Buckingham: Society for Research into Higher Education / Open University Press.

Van Ness, P.H. (ed.) (1996) *Spirituality and the Secular Quest.* London: SCM Press.

Wakefield, G. (ed.) (1983) *A Dictionary of Christian Spirituality.* London: SCM Press.

Walter, T. (1997) 'The ideology and organisation of spiritual care: three approaches.' *Palliative Medicine 11*, 21–30.

Wanless, D. (2004) *Securing Good Health for the Whole Population.* London: DoH.

Waugh, L. (1992) *Spiritual Aspects of Nursing: A Descriptive Study of Nurses' Perceptions* (unpublished PhD thesis). Edinburgh: Queen Margaret's College.

Whipp, M. (1998) 'Spirituality and the scientific mind: a dilemma for doctors.' In M. Cobb and V. Robshaw (eds) *The Spiritual Challenge of Health Care.* London: Churchill Livingstone.

Whipp, M. (2001) 'Discerning the Spirits: Theological Audit in Health Care Organisations.' In H. Orchard (ed.) *Spirituality in Health Care Contexts.* London: Jessica Kingsley Publishers.

Wilmer, H. (1997) *Spirituality at Work.* Leeds: The Leeds Institute.

World Health Organization Expert Committee (1990) *Cancer Pain Relief and Palliative Care.* Geneva: WHO.

Ziegler, J. (1998) 'Spirituality returns to the fold in medical practice.' *Journal of the American Cancer Institute 90*, 17, 1255–1257.

Further Reading

Aldridge, D. (2000) *Spirituality, Healing and Medicine: Return to the Silence.* London: Jessica Kingsley Publishers.

Church of England (2001) *A Time To Heal.* London: Church House Publishing.

Cobb, M. (2001) *The Dying Soul: Spiritual Care at the End of Life.* Buckingham: Open University Press.

Hammond, J., Hay, D., Moxon, J., Netto, B., Raban, K., Straugheir, G. and Williams, C. (1990) *New Methods in RE Teaching.* Essex: Oliver & Boyd.

Millison, M.B. (1995) 'A review of the research on spiritual care and hospice.' *The Hospice Journal 10,* 4, 3–18.

Orchard, H. (ed.) (2001) *Spirituality in Health Care Contexts.* London: Jessica Kingsley Publishers.

Rogers, J. (1989) *Adults Learning.* Milton Keynes: Open University Press.

Stanworth, R. (1997) 'Spirituality, language and depth of reality.' *International Journal of Palliative Nursing 3,* 1, 19–22.

White, G. (2000) 'An inquiry into the concepts of spirituality and spiritual care.' *International Journal of Palliative Nursing 6,* 10, 479–484.

White, G. (2002) *My Heart Sings: Learning about Spirituality in Palliative Care* (unpublished PhD thesis). Sheffield: School of Education, University of Sheffield.

Subject Index

Author Index